AN ILLUSTRATED HISTORY OF
CONTRACEPTION

AN ILLUSTRATED HISTORY OF
CONTRACEPTION

A concise account of the quest for fertility control

William H. Robertson

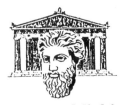

The Parthenon Publishing Group
International Publishers in Science, Technology & Education

Casterton Hall, Carnforth,
Lancs, LA6 2LA, UK

120 Mill Road, Park Ridge,
New Jersey, USA

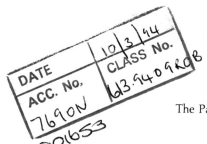

Published in the UK by
The Parthenon Publishing Group Limited
Casterton Hall, Carnforth,
Lancs, LA6 2LA, England

Published in the USA by
The Parthenon Publishing Group Inc.
120 Mill Road
Park Ridge,
New Jersey 07656, USA

Library of Congress Cataloging-in-Publication Data
Robertson, W. (William), 1921–
    An illustrated history of contraception: a concise account of the quest for fertility
control / by W. Robertson.
        p. cm.
        Bibliography: p.
    Includes index.
    ISBN 0-940813-07-6 : $45.00   .
    1. Contraception — History — Popular works. I. Title. II. Title:
History of contraception.
RG136.R56   1989   89-9339
363.9'6'09 — dc20   CIP

British Library Cataloguing in Publication Data
Robertson, W.
    An illustrated history of contraception.
    1. Man. Contraception History
    I. Title
    613.9'4'09
    ISBN 1-85070-108-3

First published 1990

Photosetting by Lasertext Ltd, Manchester
Printed in Great Britain by
Dotesios Printers Ltd, Trowbridge, Wiltshire

Dedication

In every person's life there are just a few mentors who possess rare intellect, leadership and the gift of human kindness. Robert Greenblatt would have been at home in any society; he was well read in literature, he was a distinguished historian and a world-renowned scientist and teacher. He helped me in many ways over many years. I gratefully dedicate this book to the memory of my good friend, the late Robert B. Greenblatt.

"There is a universal tendency among men to exalt the past and deprecate the present. It is hoped that the present work strikes a delicate balance."

Edward Gibbon (1737–1794)

Contents

Acknowledgements

I wish to thank many people for their help to me in the development of this book.

The late Dr Walter Fromeyer encouraged me to put pen to paper. Dr James Wilson's work on the history of contraceptive practices intrigued me. Dr Herbert Thomas gave great assistance by introducing me to several of the principals in the story, and I owe much to my old chief Dr W. Nicholson Jones and to Mrs Jean Elliot of the University of Alabama at Birmingham.

In relation to a number of the illustrations in the book, invaluable contributions were made by photographers Roy Higginbotham and Connie Scott, artist Scott Fuller, and by Ms Barbara Lyon of Abram Publishing.

Dr Richard Edgren gave me both moral and financial help, and I owe thanks also to Dr Carl Djerassi. Ortho Pharmaceutical Corporation and Syntex Laboratories Inc. gave generous help with my project. I thank my friend of many years, Dr Luigi Mastroianni, for his Preface, and appreciate the help and kindness David Bloomer and Peter Stephenson of Parthenon Publishing gave to me as a neophyte author.

My office nurse Sue Goodwin and secretaries Jimmi King, Drenda Lawley, Geri Model and Tana Park provided untiring support. Last but not least I thank Jennie my wife for her understanding, encouragement and patience.

The successful qualities in this book must be shared with several people; any errors are down to me alone.

William H. Robertson

Foreword

Down through the centuries, efforts to understand and to control fertility have been documented in almost every society. In this compendium, William Robertson has summarized this effort and, correctly, has focused on the social and biological issues that have influenced progress. It is certainly useful to reappraise the status of family planning from time to time and to place our present dilemma in historical context. The appalling fact is that, at least in terms of methodology, there have been but few major advances. With the exception of the "the pill", presently available methods have been utilized for at least a century. Some of these, such as the IUD, have been modified to make them more efficient and perhaps safer. New and imaginative approaches to the problem have been notable for their absence, recent dramatic advances in our knowledge of human reproductive biology notwithstanding.

The importance of human reproduction should be clear to all but the unthinking. Any factor which affects the reproductive potential of individuals must have broad social consequences. Paradoxically, reproductive biology, the basic underpinning for new developments in infertility treatment, equally addresses fundamental issues of family planning. As we understand how reproductive function is impaired, we are in a better position to know how to control it. There are those who take the position that the real problem in the world is not infertility but hyperfertility, and hence, efforts to treat infertility are misdirected. Yet, it is clear that we do not have methods of family planning which are appropriate and acceptable to all segments of global society, Furthermore, the search for newer and better methods of family planning has not progressed hand-in-hand with the search for newer and better methods to treat infertility.

The past two decades have witnessed dramatic breakthroughs in our understanding of human reproduction. These have lead to new and better methods to treat tubal disease, to evaluate and induce ovulation and to manage deficiencies in sperm production. The most dramatic of the recent advances has been *in vitro* fertilization. This approach has captured the imagination of the public and has done more to focus attention on the importance of basic research in human reproduction than has any other major advance. This emphasis on infertility is not misplaced when one considers its prevalence. Overall, it is estimated that one in ten couples are involuntarily infertile. In some areas of the world, and especially where population growth has been most dramatic, infertility is also endemic, occuring in as many as 20% of couples. This is largely the result of tubal disease from sexually transmitted infections. For the clinician with responsibility for individual patients, the importance of infertility is expressed best not in demographic terms but rather with reference to its impact on the lives of individuals. If we are to ask individuals to consider limiting their family size, must we not be willing to use resources to help those who do not have at least one child? Let us especially consider the devastating effect of childlessness on women, which often leads to divorce and isolation. In many societies, there are no support systems to address these issues.

Hyperfertility has an equally disasterous impact on the lives of individual women. With increasing parity, there is a progressive increase in maternal morbidity and mortality. Statistics vary tremendously from country to country. In some parts of the Third World, the lifetime risk of dying from a pregnancy-related cause is as high as one in twenty. Clearly, lack of availability of contraception has a devastating impact on the lives of those individuals. This perspective is easily lost in the overall consideration of the importance of population.

In the developed world, population growth is a non-issue. In affluent societies, the lack of availability of contraceptive measures that are safe, effective and acceptable within the cultural, social, religious and ethical frameworks of individuals has not received appropriate attention. A low priority has been given to research designed to develop better methods of family planning. Yet, contraceptive decisions, including the decision to use no contraception, must be faced by the majority of men and women of reproductive age in every society.

There is clear, albeit indirect, additional evidence that present methods are not universally acceptable and effective. Witness the high prevalence of abortion throughout the world. Many of these unwanted pregnancies result from contraceptive failure. Permanent sterilization in both the male and female has increasingly become the option of choice. The decision in favor of tubal ligation or vasectomy is often made prematurely, and increasing numbers of individuals, because of changing circumstances, now request sterilization reversal. Since present sterilization methods are designed to be permanent, methods to reverse them are complicated and are not uniformly successful.

There are many segments of society whose needs are not well served by existing methods. Particularly noteworthy in this regard are teenagers, women over 35, breastfeeding women, and those with health problems that constitute contraindications to presently available methods. Often such persons are at higher risk during pregnancy.

In the United States, a country that has made significant technological advances in other health-related areas, contraceptive development has been especially neglected. Since the development of the pill and the modern IUD almost three decades ago, no fundamentally new contraceptive has been introduced. Contraceptive development is virtually at a standstill. All but a handful of agencies and pharmaceutical companies have withdrawn from the field. Federal funding of applied contraceptive development has been declining, as has the support of private foundations. The reasons for this are complicated. They relate in part to systems of regulation and liability, but most important, to the lack of a national will.

By focusing attention on the history of contraception, we inevitably became more aware of the issues which we must face as the twenty-first century approaches. We can but hope that once again the importance of family planning will be recognized and that human reproduction will be assigned a priority commensurate with its overall impact on human well-being.

L. Mastroianni
Professor of Obstetrics and Gynecology,
University of Pennsylvania

Introduction

This is the story of man's attempt to understand and control the procreational aspect of human sexuality. The historian can trace several evolving purposes: the desire to regulate the number and uphold the quality of progeny; the need to make population growth correspond to available environment; the ambition to provide an abundant life for all.

It is not our intention that this work be an encyclopedic catalogue of all contraceptive practices; rather the purpose is to give examples of early imaginative or "magical" methods together with accounts of physiologically sound ones, whether primitive or the product of modern science.

This story includes details of brilliant observations that were undeservedly later forgotten. Our aim is to record the history of attitudes of society, governments, and religions, all of which bear upon hypotheses and discoveries. The vicissitudes of the early scientists and the later social reformers are described, and the turbulent history of the birth control movement is, hopefully, portrayed in such a manner that the heroes and heroines are given the honor due them.

In conclusion, there is an assessment of where we stand today and some suggestions as to where we might be tomorrow.

An historical essay on the development of medical knowledge must inevitably include recognition of the passions, frustrations, and sorrows of human life. Professor Arturo Castiglioni appreciated this in the preface to *The History of Medicine*. "the history has been marked by the immortal touch of genius, illuminated by the flashing light of heroism and of sacrifice, and beautified by the radiant smile of poetry. Its progress has sometimes been darkened by superstition or by dogmatism, by hatred and intolerance." All such richness is evident in the history of man's conquest of contraception.

According to Professor Arnold Toynbee in *The History of Civilization*, every state from the tribal to the industrialized considers itself an "enduring entity, each sufficient unto itself and independent of the rest of the world". He adds that historians are not immune from this sort of thinking, though the great historian Edward Gibbon shows awareness of the problem: "There is a universal tendency among men to exalt the past and deprecate the present." Each community feels itself to be the center of the universe. The more self-scrutinizing peoples have usually based their beliefs on dominant institutions whether they be the tribe, the church or parliament. Toynbee notes that historical details should not be related exclusively to their historical context. The history of contraception is certainly to be approached in the light of such observations.

Toynbee continues by remarking that the historian must study with his emotional and ethical beliefs under strict intellectual restraint. However, he goes on to say that to be completely objective is impossible. Let us bear this in mind when we study the sexual and contraceptive practices of the human race; we must view innovations within and outside their context, and we must use both detached description, and evaluation that is committed to the modern viewpoint.

This story is so varied and complex that it is necessary to generalize and compress. Not only does the account present a survey of biological and medical knowledge (or lack of it) but of sociological, scientific and religious beliefs also. There has to be careful generalization and selection under such circumstances.

Contraception and fertility have been co-existant considerations of mankind since our beginnings. Like the two faces of Janus, one looked toward the benefits of fertility and the other toward the problems of undesired progeny. In many civilizations children provided the only social security for aging or ill parents; barrenness under these circumstances was no less than a curse. In times of famine, on the other hand, too many mouths to feed could be catastrophic.

Efforts to ensure both fertility and infertility, at the times when each was wanted, were directed towards the gods and goddesses. Amulets, magic and the resources of the apothecary were in use; these all played powerful roles in pre-scientific circumstances.

Perhaps we must recognise that it could not have been otherwise when prehistoric man apparently did not perceive the function of sexual intercourse in reproduction. With no physiological knowledge available, magic and superstition filled the gap. Later, since the male semen was the only visible result of coitus, it was thought that the male contained all of the elements

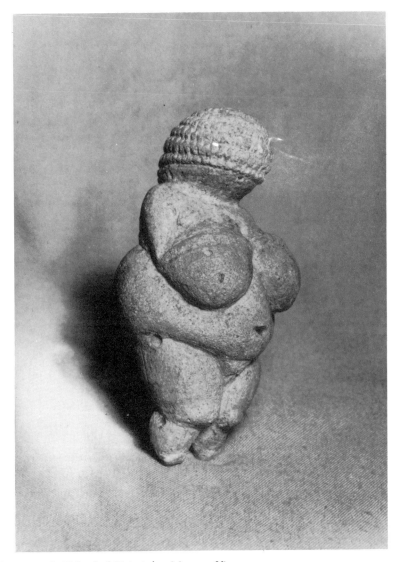

The Venus de Willendorf. Naturisches Museum, Vienna

of reproduction, and that the femal uterus served only as an incubator. One wonders how they reconciled maternal traits in the offspring!

This history of contraception must begin, therefore, in pre-literate distant historical times when attitudes to sexuality and procreation were without legitimate, as we would see it, basis in physiological knowledge.

1

Pre-literate Times

To list all the known contraceptive practices of pre-literate man would be a Herculean and inconclusive task. The selection which follows is intended to exemplify those possibly effective, those probably effective and those based on magic and superstition and therefore worthless, if considered from a physiological viewpoint alone. In all pre-literate societies the Shaman, Witch Doctor, Fetisher or the Medicine Man controlled treatment. Although they may have chanced upon some effective therapy, by and large any success was achieved by belief. Patients had a religious faith in the therapist and that brought about remedy sometimes. In considering primitive practices we must remember that pre-literate times left no records, so our conclusions, are more often than not, based on modern studies of aboriginal cultures.

First we must remind ourselves of an important factor touched upon in the Introduction namely, how often did pre-literate peoples associate coitus with conception? Clearly many contraceptive practices are going to seem bizarre if they are based on ideas which omit an understanding of the role of coitus. There are a number of theories of conception which discount intercourse. Many unphysiological notions are detailed in scholarly books such as Frazer's *The Golden Bough* and Robert Briffault's *The Mothers*. Professor Himes suggests "that a preventive technique can exist even though knowledge of the physiology of conception is very crude or even absent". After all, society had to wait for Leeuwenhoek, Swammerdam and Barry to understand the role of the sperm, the ovum and their union (see Chapter 4).

Some primitives believed that the male contribution to conception was negligible. One tribe believed that the only function of coitus was to dilate the vagina. Other societies considered paternity a social rather than a biological reality. The Euduna tribe maintained that half-white children were caused by women eating white bread rather than mating with white men.

Partial understanding of the role of coitus can be observed in some primitive peoples. The natives of Madagascar thought that after the first intercourse a woman would continue to have children whether sexually active or not. In this case no sort of contraception was practised. The population was restrained somewhat because of the rule that the husband could not cohabit with his wife for a period of three to six months after a birth. That practice was followed even after the natives became "civilized and Christian". It was also reported that some unmarried women resorted to attempt abortion but this was rare and probably not always effective since they used various herbs as abortifacients. Infanticide was also common, especially if the child was born on "unlucky days".

Most pre-literate societies resorted to abortion as a form of birth control. To kill a new-born child was not considered evil because the child was not believed to be a person until the puberty rites were performed. Infanticide was most commonly associated with individual women's ability to bring up children. It may also have been used to adjust the male-female ratio in the tribe. In some situations males will have been particularly needed because subsistence came predominantly from their hunting; in others, females provided most through their gathering function. Incidentally, Professor Himes noted that women in pre-literate societies knew all about Thomas Malthus' theory that too great a population growth endangered survival. Himes observed that the Malthus essay was "essentially a learned inductive proof of an obvious thesis long understood and long acted upon".

Since herbs have been used since ancient times, it is likely that occasionally an effective contraceptive remedy was found amongst them. An example is the use of an aqueous extract of lithospermum ruderale which has been shown to have an anovulatory effect in the experimental animal. Professor Himes in 1937 discounted all oral medication as ineffective "since no drug taken by mouth is known to Western science that will prevent conception or abort". Science was later to prove him wrong of course. One wonders how often primitive people stumbled upon something effective such as grain contaminated with ergot or the fusarium fungus which produce mycotoxins some of which have estrogenic properties, or plants of the Yam family with their now known progestational properties. The Cherokee Indians of North America are recorded as having used herbal remedies for contraception purposes. Olbrechts notes that the "Medicine Men" gave potions made from roots of spotted cowbane, to be taken orally.

The douche method has a primitive precedent in that the women of Guyana and Martinique used a solution consisting of lemon juice and an essence derived from mahogany husks. This was very probably effective since the citric acid plus the astringent action of the mahogany husks would be highly spermacidal.

Sometimes contraception was achieved by denial or restraint methods. It is known from pottery decorations that the Indians of Peru practised both oral and anal intercourse. Whether this represented deviance or sought-after sensual variety or a form of contraception must be conjectural. Coitus reservatus, or intercourse without ejaculation, was widely practised in China and it was thought to improve mind, body and potency.

There are some instances of surgical intervention to achieve contraception. The practice of subincision on the male occured amongst Australian aborigines and some peoples of the South Pacific. The operation was performed at the time of sexual maturity. The original purpose is not altogether clear. Some believe it to have been an initiation rite following which the boy became a man and part of the male community. The surgery was performed by making a slit from the urethral meatus to the scrotum. The result was that upon ejaculation the semen dribbled over the scrotum and, presumably, did not get into the vagina. An additional effect was that the man was required to squat to urinate.

Since it has been observed that these men were sometimes able to father children, some anthropologists have doubted that the intention was that of sterilization. Professor Radcliffe Brown believes that the practice of subincision was a ceremonial rite only. Professor Himes cites Dr Soloman Gandz who believes that there are veiled references to the subincision practice in the Talmud and the Bible.

In primitive societies particular sorts of manipulation of female anatomy were thought to inhibit pregnancy. One such that was at least partially effective was the production of acute retroflexion of the uterus. Apparently some of the Shamans were particularly skilled at performing this.

The aboriginal inhabitants of the Canary Islands, the Guanches, apparently did not practise contraception at all, but their response to overpopulation was grim. According to Iver Lissner, when overpopulation occurred it was decreed that all new-borns except the first be killed. Also, if a man approached a strange woman he was put to death. One method was to put the convicted in a pit. As a humane gesture he was allowed either food or water, but not both. Legend has it that one prisoner chose milk, and he lived so long that the death pit was abandoned. Why did the possessors of such great fertility become extinct? Was it war, disease, natural disaster or assimilation by neighboring Spanish or Portuguese? Since marriage between brother and sister was common perhaps genetic deterioration was the cause.

The range of contraceptive strategies amongst pre-literate peoples was thus extensive, and clearly influenced by strong micro-cultural beliefs of a non-scientific sort. As we move on to the ancient world we find more sustained and rational approaches to contraception evolving.

2

The Ancient World

As we pass from pre-literate societies to the early great civilizations the understanding of human reproduction develops. Scientific, rational understanding uneasily co-exists in many cases with residual magic. It has been said that there is nothing so practical as a good theory and nothing so bad as a false one believed to be true. Certainly, the ancient world produced theories, useful and not so useful, which contrast with the mute, instinctive practices of the pre-literate societies.

It is well to note at the outset that there was no knowledge, in ancient civilizations, of the process of ovulation. In those societies where dissection of bodies took place, understanding of the ovaries only went as far as perceiving a comparability with the male testicles. (Most translations of the word for ovaries is female testicle.) Observation of animals led many to believe that the issue of blood signaled the fertile period in humans as it does during the rut season of some animals, but there was no understanding of the discarding of an ovum which occurs at mid-cycle and not during menstruation.

Hippocrates and Pythagoras progressed as far as to hold the theory that conception occurred only through union of the male and female parts. Aristotle appears less advanced in saying that the woman was only the reservoir, and the male essence (the semen) contained all the elements necessary for reproduction. This view appears in a drama by Aeschylus: Orestes is on trial for killing his mother; Appollo testifies in his defense.

> The mother of what is called her child is no parent of it, but a nurse only of the young life that is sown in her. The parent is the male, she but the stranger, a friend who if fate spares the plant preserves it till it puts forth.

23

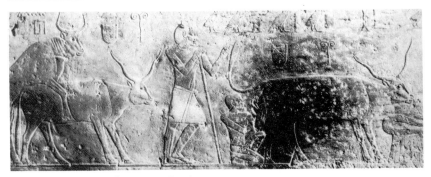

Bas relief in Saggara. (The Louvre, Paris)

ANCIENT EGYPT

The first step in the application of any successful contraceptive is the recognition of the relationship between coitus and conception. There is an ancient Bas relief in Saggara (Northern Egypt) that clearly depicts a bull mounting a cow followed by the delivery of a calf (see illustration). Despite this apparent insight, magic remained a vital part of contraceptive practice in ancient Egypt. There were glimpses of scientifically derived methods confirmed by trial and error, but such glimpses were accompanied by persisting recourse to sorcery and superstition.

According to Professor Himes the oldest medical prescription for the prevention of conception is contained in the *Petri Papyrus*, discovered at Kahûn in 1889. It was written during the reign of Amenemhat III, of the Twelfth Dynasty (c. 1850 BC). The translator, F. Griffith, characterized most of the prescriptions as "obvious quackery". Professor Himes takes issue, however, with that assessment and cites several examples that seem to have logic. One consists of a paste-like substance, containing crocodile dung, used as a pessary. Another was a pessary consisting of honey and natron (sodium carbonate) and another which included a gum-like material for intra vaginal use. All these would tend to have some spermicidal as well as barrier effect. The Egyptians were much taken with the use of dung; they first used crocodile and later substituted elephant. Whether or not the PH factor had any effect is conjectural; possibly the sticky material had some mechanical effect also.

The *Ebers Papyrus* was written over an extended period of time. The last additions were probably around 1550 BC. The most effective preparation described was the use of tips from the acacia tree which contain gum arabic. When fermentation takes place, lactic acid is liberated (an ingredient of most

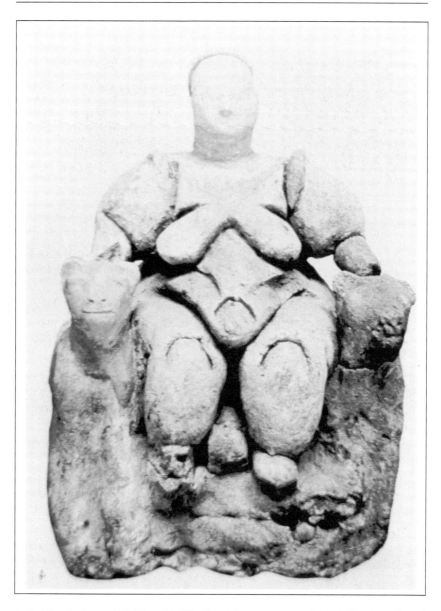

Seated female figure (c. 6500–5700 BC). Found in excavations of Catal Hüyük in Central Turkey. Thought to be a fertility goddess giving birth. (Archaeological Museum, Ankara)

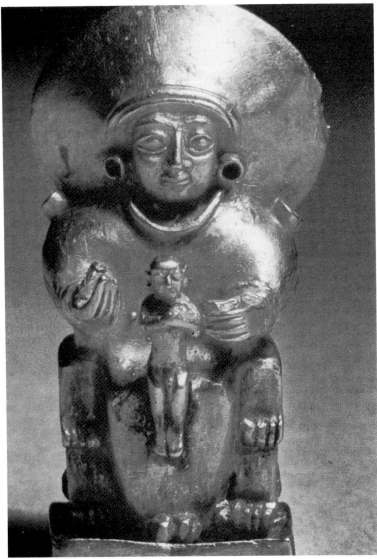

A golden fertility icon. Mesopotamian Madonna (c. 1400–1200 BC). (Collection Norbert Schimmel, New York)

contraceptive jellies today). This is combined with honey which acts as an adhesive and barrier in addition to the spermicidal effect of the lactic acid. The Egyptians also used a pre-coital fumigation technique with, presumably, a herb of some kind.

The *Berlin Papyrus* (c.1300 BC) was possibly copied from an earlier one. It is difficult to interpret, although eight sections seem to deal with contraception. Himes characterizes these as "quasi-magical".

After studious consideration Professor Himes summarizes the three papyri as follows: "The Petri is partially effective; the Ebers is better because it combines physical and chemical features; the Berlin is magical and worthless".

As a general comment, Professor Himes considers it unusual that olive oil, widely used in ancient Egypt as a cosmetic aid, in cooking and for the local treatment of wounds, is not mentioned as being of use in contraception.

It seems apparent that the upper class of Egyptians had some understanding of reproductive physiology. In painting and sculpture, the nobility are depicted with the women thin and beautiful, and accompanied by just a few children. According to the Greek historian, Strabo (63BC–AD21), ovariotomies were commonly performed on the higher classes. One would like to know the technique used and the complications encountered. Perhaps this information along with much else was lost when the famous library at Alexandria was destroyed. They may have felt that surgery was no more dangerous than was pregnancy and delivery. But, as everyone now knows, there are hidden dangers in pregnancy. In fact, it is only in modern times that parturition has become overwhelmingly safe. Before the modern era a pregnant woman was at considerable risk.

The famous (or infamous) Queen Cleopatra provides occasion for interesting consideration of contraceptive methods in Ancient Egypt. It has seemed obvious to historians that she knew some method of contraception because she was only pregnant three times. She had a son by Caesar, and twins and a son by Mark Anthony. Shirley Green postulates that she was very likely familiar with Aristotle's *Historica Animalum* in which it was suggested that the cervix be covered with oil of cedar or ointment of lead or with frankincense and olive oil.

ANCIENT GREECE

Medicine and its relationship to population growth was clearly important amongst the ancient Greeks. We find that the topic has a place within the rich mythological network of the culture, contributing to the correct impression that this civilization pushed forward the evolution of medicine as it did similarly in other areas of knowledge.

Askelepios was a Greek physician who practised medicine with his two sons, Machaon and Podaleiros. They were extremely proficient particularly in the treatment of battle wounds, and their ability to save lives was so great that the population of Hades, the Underworld, was diminishing. This disturbed Pluto, the Lord of Hades, who complained to Zeus who responded by having Askelepios killed by a thunderbolt. Legends developed portraying Askelepios as a god; it was thought that no one of pedestrian ancestry could be so great. The theory evolved that he was the son of Apollo and a mortal mother Koronis. Obstetrical complications caused her death and Askelepios was brought into the world by what we would term a *post-mortem* Caesarian section.

A cult of skilled physicians developed called the "Askelepiads"; their emphasis was on diagnosis of disease rather than the favorable relationship (or otherwise) of the patient to the gods. These physicians did not base their work on the belief that illness was a sign of deistic wrath. In the later period of ancient Greek civilization literal belief in the gods was not adhered to in general, and certainly in connection with medicine we see a significant shift from superstition to early scientific observation and method.

Soranos (98–138BC) was the most accomplished gynecologist of antiquity. He makes a definite distinction between contraception and abortion. Departing from the teachings of Hippocrates, whom we shall discuss later, he believes that abortion is sometimes indicated when it is dangerous for the mother because of a small pelvis, tumors or other health problems, but never because of adultery, to preserve beauty or other frivolous reasons.

Soranos advocates gymnastics such as pelvic movements, holding the breath at the time of ejaculation, getting up and sitting down with bent knees and inducing sneezing. More significantly, he advises precoital application to the cervix of oil or honey or cedar gum or opabalsam either together or mixed with ceruse (white lead) or with an ointment which is prepared with myrtle oil and ceruse, or with alum, or galbanum in wine. He also suggests the introduction of soft wool into the mouth of the womb before coitus. Another pessary is described using pine bark, *rhus coriaria*, wine and wool, or pulverized pomegranate mixed with gall nut, or pulp of dry figs with natron (sodium carbonate). To his considerable credit he says that the use, of amulets is "delusive"; clearly he had the resources to resist superstition. While the preparations listed so far would have had some degree of contraceptive effect, some of Soranos' others must have been of no use at all. He advises that one swallow cyrenaic sap juice, or mix opopanax, cyrenaic sap and the juice of rue and make a pill with wax to be swallowed with watered wine. He mentions potions of myrrh and white pepper, a draught of one obol of hedge mustard seeds and a mixture of

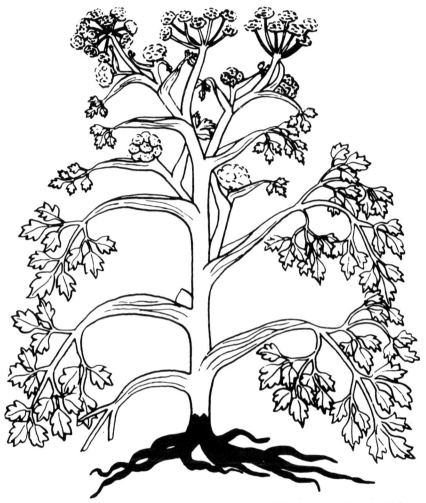

Panas Heraklios, today called Ferula opopanax or Opopanax hispidus (Giant fennel). *Medicina Magica.* (Courtesy of Akademische Druck-u. Verlagsanstalt, Graz, Austria)

spondylium and sour honey!

Most intriguing is the report that Soranos belonged to the "Methodist" sect, a group whose approach to science was painstaking and methodical. It would be interesting to know more of this group's procedures and achievements. The existence of such a sect is further instance of scientific objectivity making inroads into ancient superstition and mythology. Soranos' writings on contraception reveal an encyclopedic knowledge for his time

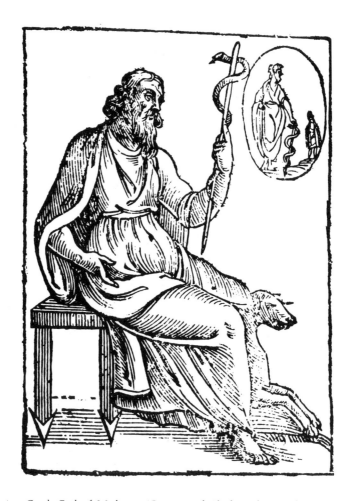

Askelepios, Greek God of Medicine. (Courtesy of Akademische Druck-u. Verlagsanstalt, Graz, Austria)

plus an originality and a rationality of approach. Despite his great intellect he fell into the common error concerning the "safe period", which error persisted until the timing of ovulation was discovered. He considered the "dangerous" times of the cycle to be just before and just after the menstrual period. As we now know, it is in the mid cycle that ovulation occurs.

So Soranos strikes us as showing some "modern" views; he dismisses amulets and the like; he has interest in discovering successful pessaries; he recommends coitus interruptus and douching, and has moral reservations

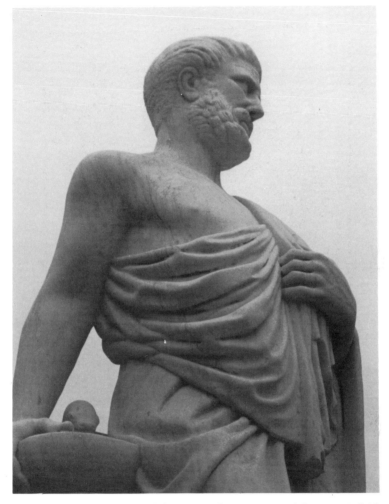

Hippocrates. Sculpture by Kostos Nikolaou Georgakas. (Courtesy of the Lister Hill Library and the University of Alabama at Birmingham)

concerning abortion; above all, perhaps, he apparently sets value on scientific method.

Mention must be made of a third major figure, Hippocrates. He offered a number of ideas on contraception in his treatise *On the Nature of Women*. For cervicitis he recommended use of a tampon containing misy, but this cannot have had contraceptive intention since it was to be removed prior to intercourse. He makes veiled references to the value of coitus interruptus, mentioned too the simple procedure of using the fingers to wipe out the vagina. Abortion was unacceptable to him: "I shall never prescribe a phtorion".

Aristotle, on the other hand, condoned abortion but before "sense and life have begun". How he determined this is not recorded. He considered infanticide cruel and immoral.

Hippocrates noted that fat women tended to be infertile and, according to Haeser, he advocated weight gain for its contraceptive effect. This was a shrewd observation characteristic of the great Greek physician. It may be that the idea came to him because he noticed that the Scythian women were both corpulent and relatively infertile. Hippocrates' observation was all the more remarkable since there was no knowledge at the time of the endocrine system. When others in the ancient world came to associate corpulence with infertility the idea became part of folk tradition.

THE HEBREWS

The Bible offers many indications as to attitudes taken by the Hebrews as far as population and contraception are concerned. Professor Robert Greenblatt in his most entertaining and erudite book *Search the Scriptures* mentions the practice of sexual continence when population growth would be inappropriate.

> "Defraud ye not the other, except it be with consent for a time, that ye may give yourselves to fasting and prayer; and come together again, that satan tempt you not for your incontinency".
>
> (1 Corinthians 7:5)

Professor Greenblatt asks the following questions. Is temporary abstinence a satisfactory approach to contraception in love and marriage? Can man harness the "creative force" to avoid the world catastrophe of the population explosion?

We shall subsequently note the controversial practice of coitus interruptus and the sin of Onan and Er. Even though some rabbis condoned coitus interruptus it continued to carry a stigma. During the captivity in Egypt, the Hebrews learned the use of barrier pessaries. The sponge "makk" was adopted from the Egyptian lint. Mixtures of acacia and honey were frequently used.

The sponge or pessary was considered more acceptable to later rabbis because the man was considered the one commanded to propagate the race,

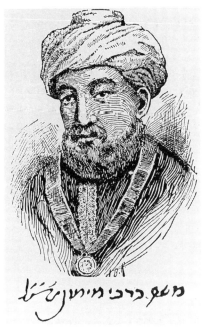

Maimonides. Philosopher and physician compiler of a pharmacopeia — including mention of drugs which "sterilize". Engraved portrait with facsimile autograph. (Courtesy of New York Academy of Medicine, New York)

and since the woman was under no such compulsion she was free to use the sponge. This seems to be disreputable "passing of the buck".

Moses' injunction to the Children of Israel to be fruitful specified the time for love.

> "And if a woman have an issue of her blood she shall be unclean. But if she be cleansed of her issue, then she shall number to herself seven days and after that she shall be clean."
>
> Levitivus 15: 19–25

This clearly demonstrates that the ancient Hebrews were well aware of the fertile period. By contrast, the Egyptians were under the sway of sorcery. Moses banned the use of sorcery altogether by the children of Israel.

Jesus of Nazareth was intriguingly silent on the subject of contraception. Presumably his views were those shared by the majority of the followers of Judaism. The emphasis was on fruitfulness.

ANCIENT CHINA

Professor Himes found the study of Chinese customs frustrating because it was difficult, if not impossible, to separate contraceptive from abortifacient intentions. Some of the prescriptions date from 2000 BC. They share qualities with other ancient therapies: magic, sorcery and superstition. One popular method was to swallow sixteen tadpoles fried in quicksilver! A less extraordinary recipe calls for the use of a leaven made of wheat flour, kidney beans, *polygonum flaccidum,* and apricot kernels. The use of apricot kernels is interesting because of the present-day belief by some that a substance found therein is cancerocidal (Laertrill).

It is well to remember that ancient remedies which appear bizarre to us now sometimes represent a sound biochemical application. In areas when there were few methods of isolating individual substances, a vehicle substance, usually complex and organic was accepted. Perhaps the practice is not wholly unfamiliar even now; we use "royal jelly", cod-liver oil and the like, the difference being we know and evaluate the constituent substances.

The Chinese also practised coitus reservatus. It was thought that the more times one could engage in coitus without emission the more potent one would become. The belief was that "the essence" found its way to the brain, resulting in improvement in many ways (mind, body and estate).

Before leaving consideration of the ancient world we need to comment in general upon two factors which bear upon the issue of contraception: population control and consanguinity. Most of the ancients were interested in maintaining a population density sufficient to support the economy. Too many mouths to feed would obviously present a problem. In most cases, of course, this was controlled by natural causes such as disease, accidents, war and so forth. Aristotle, Plato, Hesiod, and Polybius were all concerned with population problems. Jesus, Zenocrates and Lycurgus favored the one child family. Plato believed that the age span for reproductive life should be regulated legally — for the male 30–35 and 20–40 for the female.

In general, the Hebrews responded to the biblical direction "Be fruitful and multiply and replenish the Earth" (Genesis). But by the time of Alexander the Great (330 BC) Palestine was overcrowded and agriculture was no longer able to support the people. The response to this challenge was emigration and the abandonment of the practice of polygamy. Wherever they went in the world, however, they returned to the original emphasis on fertility just as long as conditions were favorable.

Advantageous population control also involved attention to the number of non-productive, congenitally defective people in society. In this regard, genetic dangers, particularly those related to incest were recognized in different cultures at different times. Quite possibly the danger of inbreeding was first observed in domesticated animals. The value of hybrid vigor was recognized in many cultures, and attitudes towards contraception where consanguinity was a threat became strong as a consequence.

Religious taboos and legal restrictions regarding inbreeding had a definite but limited influence on population. This is true for two reasons: first, marital partners usually came from the same vicinity (often they were raised only yards apart) consequently kinship was common; secondly, among the higher echelons of society the importance of family outweighed the dangers of inbreeding. Modern examples are well known in royal families, i.e. hemophilia in Queen Victoria's progeny, porphyria in George III (and presumably in Mary Queen of Scots), as well as the numerous inherited defects suffered by the Habsburgs.

The ancient Hebrews were particularly concerned with incest. Forbidden were blood relatives such as sister, half sister, mother and aunt. Strangely the prohibition extended to persons who did not share common genes such as aunts by marriage and even godchildren. Nieces who did share genes were permitted. Clearly the Hebrews did not understand the whole picture of inheritance.

Similarly the Koran offers medically illogical rules. In addition to a list of blood relatives, also proscribed were stepdaughters, or their daughters, daughters-in-law or two sisters.

Perhaps some of these restrictions were imposed more for domestic peace than either for population control or the quality of the offspring!

During the latter part of the ancient period there occurred an event that was destined profoundly to affect science during the oncoming Middle Ages. We refer to the conversion of the Roman Emperor Constantine (388–337) to Christianity. He made it the official religion of the empire and adopted the sacred Chi-Rho (☧) seal. The stage was thus set for the eventual domination of European society by the Roman Catholic Church with some interesting moral and anti-scientific influences on the subject of contraception and birth control.

3

The Middle Ages

The liberty of thought that had prevailed during the flowering of Greek culture allowed free expression by the philosophers and scientists. According to Durant they were "unafraid in the presence of religious or political taboos and boldly subpoenaed every creed and institution to appear before the judgement seat of reason". This liberty was drastically curtailed during the Middle Ages in Europe by the dominant Roman Catholic Church.

During the Middle Ages there was a difference in attitudes between the Islamic world and Europe concerning contraception and the dissemination of medical and scientific knowledge. In Islam, physicans were orientated toward science and were unencumbered by religious restraint. The scientific giants during this period were Aëtios, Al-Razi (Rhazes), Ali ibn Abba, Avicenna, Ismail Jurjani, Ibn al-Jami and Ibn al-Batar.

It is important to remember that Islamic religious law did not forbid contraception nor was abortion against religious doctrine.

THE ISLAMIC WORLD

Aëtios of Amida (527–565)

Aetios ranks in brilliance with Soranos. As contraceptives, he recommends pessaries similar to those ascribed to Soranos, using astringents, oil, honey and resins to be applied to the cervix. One would expect these to be relatively effective. After his learned description of barrier and spermicidal preparations he goes on, however, to recommend amulets, one described as myrtle and berries soaked in the milk of a she ass and wrapped in the skin of a hare; the amulet must not be allowed to touch the ground. Another contained the milk tooth of a child or a marble, and was to be worn near the anus.

Al-Razi (Rhazes) (died c. 923–927)

Abu Bakr Muhammed ibn Zakariya Al-Razi was born near Tehran, Persia, during the mid-ninth century, the exact dates of his birth and death being unknown. Rhazes is often compared to Hippocrates because of his clear and practical approach to medicine. His writings were encyclopedic and included a history of contraception. In his *Quintessence of Experience* he describes contraceptive techniques:

> "Occasionally it is very important that the semen should not enter the womb, as for instance when there is danger to the woman in pregnancy, or, if it has entered, that it should come out again. There are several ways of preventing its entrance. The first is that at the time of ejaculation the man withdraw from the woman so that the semen does not approach the os uteri. The second way is to prevent ejaculation, a method practised by some. A third method is to apply to the os uteri, before intromission, some drug which blocks the uterine aperture or which expels the semen and prevents conception, such as pills or pessaries."

Rhazes emphasizes the usefulness of vaginal suppositories of which he lists 15. He also recommends blockage of the passage of semen, presumably by compressing the urethra. Also he includes techniques to produce abortion. In addition, he advocates useless fumigations and potions and discusses methods of expelling the semen by violent movements. If this is unsuccessful and conception occurs, he advises probing the uterus to produce abortion.

In Rhazes' treatise, as in much of ancient medicine, the rational and the what now appears ridiculous are mingled. Salt is an effective spermicide but would have to be used pre-coitally for maximum effectiveness. Male acceptance of this substance could be a problem, as the male urethra is much more sensitive than the female vagina, and so burning might be a deterrent. Cabbage or willow leaf suppositories were probably partially effective since the cervical canal would be blocked. Animal membrane used as a vaginal condom would also be relatively effective. This latter idea is not new; certain African women have, since time immemorial, used the hollowed-out okra pod as a vaginal sac. Compared with these at least partially effective prescriptions, Rhazes also makes some bizarre suggestions. Efforts to dislodge the semen by acrobatic exercise by the female are recommended. There is even faith in magic numbers; if a woman jumps backwards seven times some contraceptive effect will apparently be achieved.

According to Professor Himes, Rhazes's *Quintessence of Experience* has not survived in its entirety. The manuscript is incomplete with partial Latin translations being extant. Rhazes was a very great physician inferior only

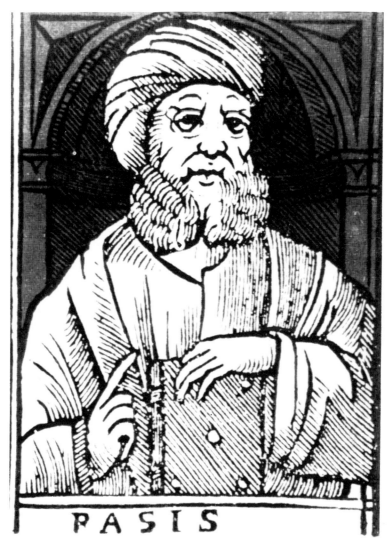

PASIS

Rhazes. Woodcut. (Courtesy of the New York Academy of Medicine, New York)

to Soranos and Aëtios. He clearly felt that a discussion of contraception was essential and certainly not obscene.

Ali ibn Abba – The Royal Book (Liber Regius)

The Royal Book, written in AD 994, included a treatise, "The Perfection of the Art." The author was one of the greatest physicians of the eastern caliphate and the following paragraphs are from Chapter 28 which considers contraception measures (translated by Professor Norman Himes):

> "As to the remedies which prevent conception, it ought to be a duty not to mention them (in this treatise) in order that they might not be used by certain ill-famed women; it is nevertheless indispensable to administer them to those women who have a small uterus, or to those suffering from a disease which would render gravidity so dangerous that the patient might die during parturition. Except for women in such predicaments the physician should never impart contraceptive information to women, nor should he ever prescribe remedies calculated to suppress the menses, nor remedies for causing abortion, except to trustworthy women inasmuch as all these remedies kill the embryo and expel it".

Conception will be prevented if women insert rock salt in the vagina during coitus, or induce the man to anoint his penis with the same material, or with tar; or if the woman insert the flowers and seed of cabbage and the juice of rue during or after coitus, or carries (in her vagina) the rennet of rabbits (membrane of stomach) or the leaves of the weeping willow.

Ibn Abba's *Royal Book* appears more systematic and concise than Rhazes's and more practical than that of Avicenna.

Ibn Sī-nā – The Canon of Avicenna (Quanun) (980–1037)

Avicenna was the most renowned physician and philosopher of medieval Islam. His monumental *Canon* enjoyed unprecedented influence from 1100 to 1500. He was gifted with high intellect but was no ascetic; his indulgence in the pleasures of the flesh led to ill health and eventually caused his death.

Avicenna was a man of many parts, a Leonardo of the Islamic world. Although his contraceptive prescriptions seem slightly less reasonable than those of his predecessors, Soranos and Aëtios, his accomplishments were great including those of encylopedist, philosopher, physician and astronomer. Acceptance of his work was as complete as was that of Galen later; this attitude discouraged original scientific inquiry on the part of others of his time. His authority was almost equal to that which Aristotle had wielded.

Avicenna's recommendation for contraception were:

1. Avoidance of simultaneous orgasm;
2. Practice of coitus interruptus;
3. Avoidance of intercourse at a time likely to result in conception; (Since ovulation physiology was not understood, this was a guess.)
4. Violent jumping by the woman to dislodge semen;

5. Insertion of tar into the vagina and/or anointing the penis with tar or oil and white lead;
6. Insertion of leaves and seed mixed with tar into the vagina;
7. Insertion of pessaries made of colocynth, mandrake, sulfur, iron dross and cabbage seed mixed with oil;
8. Smearing the penis with sweet oil before coitus.

Avicenna was well ahead of his time because most of his contraceptive

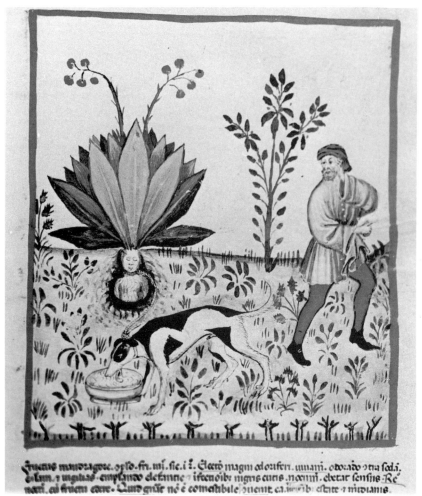

Mandrake. Tacuinum sanitates. (Courtesy of Akademische Druck-u. Verlagsanstalt, Graz, Austria)

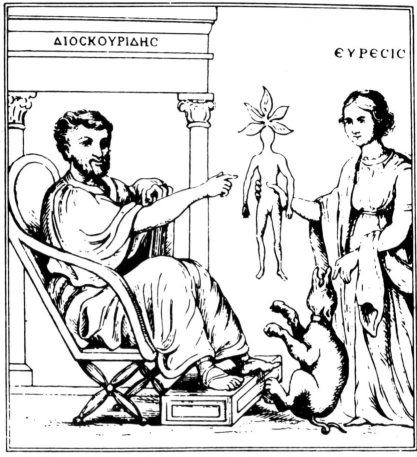

ΔΙΟCΚΟΥΡΙΔΗC

ΕΥΡΕCΙC

Dioskurides, reputedly the greatest herbalist of the ancient world, depicted discoursing on mandrake. (Courtesy of Akademische Druck-u. Verlagsanstalt, Graz, Austria)

prescriptions were sound. Despite this he relied on magical numbers i.e. for the woman to jump back seven or nine times. (Forward jumping in fact causes retention of the semen and is bad.) Also, he favored the post-coital rather than the pre-coital use of suppositories. Medical historian, Fielding Garrison, comments that Avicenna's overall influence on medieval medicine was not beneficial because he was apparently responsible for the "pernicious idea that ratiocination is better than firsthand (observation)."

Ismail Jurjani

This Persian physician wrote *The Treasure of Medicine*, which was probably the first encyclopedic work written in Persian rather than Arabic. The following translation is by Dr Cyril Algood of Wareham, Dorset, England.

> "Whenever a woman is of tender years or suffers from weakness of the
> bladder, or whenever there is a fear that pregnancy will bring on some
> ailment such as incontinence of urine, uterine erosions, and so forth, it
> is thought good to use some plan to prevent pregnancy."

He further suggested that simultaneous orgasm be avoided and that the
couple should come apart rapidly, following which the woman should have
a good shake and provoke sneezing in order to dislodge the semen. The
idea has logic, but as a technique lacked effectiveness! As a pre-coital
precaution, he advised that the woman eat cabbage or drink sweet basil. He
also prescribed a pessary consisting of colocynth pulp, bryony, iron scoria,
sulfur, scammony and cabbage seed mixed with tar. Most of these
prescriptions, as we have seen date back to Soranos, Avicenna or Ali ibn
Abba.

Ibn al-Jami

A Jewish physician at the court of Sultan Saladin, Al-Jami practised medicine
from 1171 to 1193. His principal work was *The Book of Right Conduct
Regarding the Supervision of the Soul and Body*. For contraception, he
recommended anointing the penis with onion juice prior to intercourse. He
also mentioned tampons impregnated with peppermint, pennyroyal or leek
seeds. In addition to these generally effective contraceptive prescriptions,
he advised such ineffective methods as eating beans on an empty stomach.

Ibn al-Batar (d. 1248)

This individual apparently ushered in a period of decline in the effectiveness
of Islamic contraceptive advice. Primarily a pharmacologist and a compiler
of prescriptions, he listed some 1400 items, including those recommended
to produce abortion, and others with aphrodisiac properties.

CHRISTIAN EUROPE

European customs and behavior were profoundly influenced during the
Middle Ages by the Roman Catholic Church, particularly in matters relating
to sexuality, marriage and reproduction. The teachings of St Augustine
(354–430) had a marked effect on all theological thought and, consequently,

on church approval of the practical aspects of life. Augustine defended the ideals of Christianity through his great works, *Confessions* and *The City of God*, both basically autobiographical. One goal of his writings was to define the purpose of marriage, and in his tract, "Marriage and Concupiscence", he condemned contraception even for married persons.

St Thomas Aquinas (1225–1274), who became the chief spokesman for the Roman Catholic Church during the Middle Ages, adopted many of Augustine's teachings. Aquinas, whose approach to problems was more philosophical than scientific, sought to reconcile Aristotle's theories with Muslim and Christian ethics. Aristotle had reported on contraceptive techniques without expressing either approval or disapproval of the practice. Aquinas, expressing most of his viewpoints in his most important work, *Summa Theologica*, says, concerning contraception, "Insofar as the generation of offspring is impeded, it is a vice against nature which happens in every carnal act from which generation cannot follow. Whenever pleasure is the chief motive for the marriage act, it is a mortal sin; when it is an indirect motive, it is a venial sin, and when it spurns pleasure altogether and is displeasing, it is wholly void of venial sin." Such an attitude, to most minds altogether contrary to human nature, is not likely to lead to marital harmony.

This Thomistic doctrine became the official stand of the Roman Catholic Church, thus stifling any inquiry concerning reproduction. Scientific and political thought as a whole was held back by Aquinas' influence. The sentiments of Aquinas were echoed by Dante in the *Inferno*, when he said that carnal sinners are doomed to torment; such people are condemned for subordinating reason to lust.

In England, the early Roman occupation of Britain had to a degree Romanized the native population. This meant that some of the contraceptive knowledge possessed by the Romans had been acquired by the Britons. The use of goats' bladders as condoms, coitus interruptus, use of vaginal tampons and the observed sterility of eunuchs can be traced back to Roman influence. Some practices were apparently not recorded in the literature. For instance, the Leech books, written between AD 900 and AD 950, do not mention contraceptive techniques, although 41 crafts (sections) were devoted to the related areas of obstetrics and gynecology.

Albert the Great (1193–1280)

Albert, born in Swabia in Bavaria, was a Dominican philosopher characterized by Professor Himes as a weaker theologian but a better scientist than St

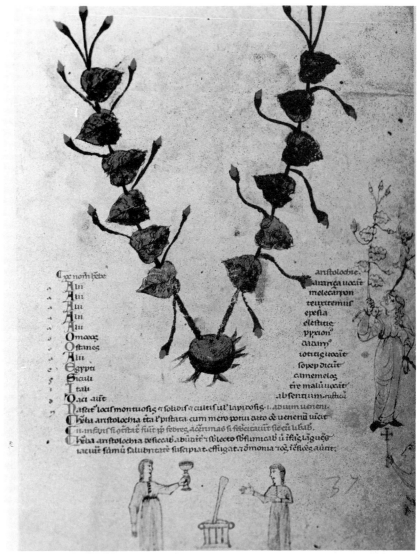

Birthwort. Used in midwifery. (Courtesy of Akademische Druck-u. Verlagsanstalt, Graz, Austria)

Thomas. He wrote encyclopedic treatises on science, philosophy and theology. His contributions to contraception were essentially based on magic and thus valueless. An example of this is his statement that if a woman spat 3 times into the mouth of a frog or if she ate bees, she would not become pregnant. He also recorded the belief that if a woman remained passive during intercourse she would not become pregnant, and this belief was shared by other cultures, including the Chinese. Albert listed a number of drugs and plant substances which could be used to prevent pregnancy, among these, drinking sabine (liquid from *juniperus sabina*) was popularly believed to be effective as a contraceptive.

Since Thomism stifled scientific investigation, the more intelligent of the populace consulted the classical writers of Greece and Rome. In spite of ecclesiastic repression, there was some advance in medical thought although it was characterized by Castiglioni as occurring "feebly and slowly". One of the more advanced centers of learning was the School of Salerno, and the most important medical document produced there was *De Aegritudinum Curatione*. This anonymous collection of writings was derived principally from Arabic medical texts, which probably accounts for its occasional sound reasoning. The chapter on the genitalia includes contraceptive measures, aphrodisiacs and abortifacients. Since the members of the School of Salerno carried out their own anatomical dissections, they were able to refute many of the errors of Galen. The initial brilliance of the School ended when it was taken over by ecclesiastics.

Arnold of Villanova

This prolific writer on most current medical topics was born near Valencia in 1235. He was an independent thinker who did not hesitate to contradict the dicta of such esteemed authorities as Galen and Avicenna. He revived Soranus' belief that drinking water in which smith's forceps had been cooled would produce sterility. While he professed disbelief in magic and sorcery, his writings contain many superstitions.

The teachings of St Thomas left no doubt concerning the Church's stand towards contraception. Although, as has been noted, the Middle Ages in Europe were characterized by domination of the Church, nevertheless as Professor Himes writes, "It is abundantly clear that even in the Middle Ages, the era of greatest dominance of the Church, when Europe was culturally unified and dominated by custom almost to the point of stagnation, the Church never succeeded in preventing the application of contraceptive knowledge." Nevertheless, there were great impediments to the advancement of science. An eighteenth-century assessment was made sardonically by Alexander Pope who said that "The monks have finished what the Goths began".

It should be noted to the credit of the Church that, despite the backwardness of medicine during the Middle Ages, hospital growth accelerated under Church sponsorship.

Whether or not the primitive and magical, alternating at times with the practical contraceptive methods, affected the natality figures is in doubt, due to lack of records on the subject. Possibly physicians of the time knew more than the folk remedies which have been recorded. It is, however, most likely that contraception did not affect population to any great extent.

Frater Rudolphus

This writer of the fourteenth century in his manuscript, *De Officio Cherubyn* catalogs many superstitions concerning pregnancy prevention. He felt that belief in such methods compromised religious belief, and he admonished priests to be aware of such beliefs and practices in order to combat them. He observed that many women believed that they could limit the number of children that they would have by sitting on as many fingers. In this context, one finds many records of the use of the fingers in ritualistic contraceptive superstition. Hovorka reported that Serbian women would dip fingers in the first bath water of an infant; the number of fingers dipped represented the number of years of desired sterility. Brides in the Baltic island of Öland touched the cervix with as many fingers as they desired children. The reason for the widespread use of fingers is not known. Perhaps it was merely a method of counting – a physiological symbol, or was it a phallic symbol? The present-day obscene use of "the finger" is clearly phallic in intent.

When one compares the contraceptive information found in the writings of Avicenna and Rhazes of the Islamic World with the information in those of Albert the Great or Arnold of Villanova, it is apparent that Islamic knowledge and writings on the subject were markedly more advanced than were those in Europe.

CHINA IN THE MIDDLE AGES

The history of contraception in China during the Middle Ages is obscure. When Professor Himes wrote his classic book a number of sinologists were unable to cite any pertinent references. One reason is that the Chinese put a premium on large families, especially sons. Only the diligent searches of Michael Hagerty of the United States Department of Agriculture and the

University of California produced any information. He found the earliest reference to the subject in *A Thousand Gold Prescriptions* written by Sun Ssu-mo, who died in AD 695. It is possible to infer from this work that abortions and infanticide had been performed since more ancient times.

The early history of contraception in Japan remains a mystery, but because of the cultural ties between China and Japan, it is assumed that their contraceptive practices were similar. Professor Himes points out that the tradition of family solidarity and the desire to limit the number of births is not new.

A German anthropologist, Schedel, reported in 1909 that a "helmet" made of tortoise shell for the penis glans (kabuto-gato) was widely used in Japan in early days. It was reputed to give the woman much pleasure, but no mention is made of the male partner.

CONTRACEPTION AND THE STATUS OF WOMEN IN THE EUROPEAN MIDDLE AGES

In most medieval societies the female was regarded as little more than a beast of burden and a sexual object. Aristotle said that the last thing that

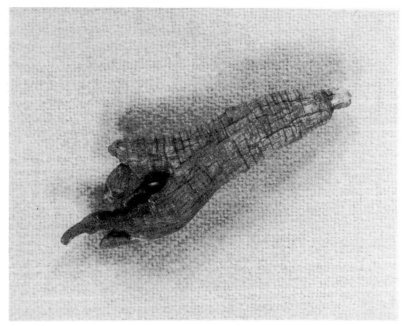

Ginseng. Panax ginseng — China. Thought to resemble the human body, it is   used extensively in medicine for many indications including impotence and as an aphrodisiac

would be civilized would be woman. This "evaluation" was superseded by the cult of the Virgin and the emergence of chivalric love. Since contraception has usually been the responsibility of the woman, an elevation in her status was important, especially in its effect on family planning.

The age of chivalry which evolved from feudalism reached its peak in the 12th and 13th centuries. One of its principal characteristics was the elevation in the status of women. The guilt of Eve attributed to women in general gave way to the cult of the Virgin, which led to the glorification of womanhood. Expression of this attitude is found in such literature as versions of the Arthurian legends like the epics of Chretien de Troyes and in the Roman de la Rose. These writings greatly influenced contemporary social behavior as well as subsequent literature.

The sainthood of Mary raised the status of women and removed much of the taint of original sin from them; however, carnal desire endured as a problem. The chivalric knight was ideally expected not to feel carnal love, but rather a purer, platonic affection for the object of his admiration. But at the center of the Arthurian legends lies the illicit relation between Guinevere and Lancelot. In actual life many husbands of admired women distrusted their wives' faithfulness and insisted on the use of the chastity belt. Then as now, when sexual habits are in question, one must consider "what is" rather than "what should be".

CONCLUSION

When one evaluates the contraceptive therapies of earlier scientists and physicians, one must, in Descartes' words, see not only copper and glass but sometimes the gold and diamonds of insight. It is remarkable that early physicians did as well as they did with their imperfect knowledge of reproductive physiology. Some very effective barrier methods were recommended and used. Although we tend to be shocked or amused at their sometimes vile oral preparations, the idea of an effective medication to prevent pregnancy was destined after much trial and failure to come to fruition in our time with "the Pill".

The efforts of the Thomists to suppress what was conceived as a vice — that is, contraception — were not, in their thinking, unreasonable. The preceding eras had been characterized by sexual licentiousness; the orgies of Rome had not been forgotten neither had the wild behavior of the gods of ancient Greece and Rome. St Thomas was leading a pervasive fight against paganism and superstition. He longed for a return to the teachings of Christ and the Pauline doctrines. He believed that any sexual enjoyment was sinful, but since orgasm in the male is essential for ejaculation, it was condoned for married men, but only for the purpose of procreation. Although the man had to reach a climax, it was acceptable only if he did *not* enjoy it. The woman should remain passive during intercourse. That Aquinas' influence suppressed scientific inquiry has to be judged very unfortunate.

In Europe the curfew that the church placed on science was to be reversed during the Age of Enlightenment in the 18th and 19th centuries.

4

The Renaissance and the Early Development of Reproductive Physiology

During the Middle Ages, all nature was explained in deistic terms. Clearly, scientific development could not occur until unrestricted investigation was possible. Scientists did not lack intelligence, but its exercise was hampered by fear and consequently lack of resolve. Immanuel Kant wrote in 1784 that man in the Middle Ages had been living in a non-age which was only overcome by what he termed "sapere aude" — dare to know. Scientists of the Enlightenment argued that the increased understanding of science would ultimately provide knowledge of God's plan. Just as the scriptures provided God's word, a study of natural science would provide knowledge of his works.

The event initiating the Enlightenment was the rediscovery of the classics of Greece and Rome. This was followed by critical analyses by original thinkers. The fall of Constantinople had led to an influx of middle eastern immigrants into Southern Italy, and it was their presence which led to a revived interest in literature, art and science. Independent thought, previously checked, began timidly to reassert itself. Near the end of the 15th century the laity gained control of the universities so that, at last, the faculties were freed, to an extent, from ecclesiastic restraint. Unfettered investigation, long forgotten or practised surreptitiously, again became part of the medical curriculum. In addition, the new art of printing made wide distribution of medical texts possible, and those yearning for knowledge no longer needed to be near the great libraries. Arturo Castiglioni characterized this period as the "Dawn of scientific liberty and the beginning of biological and

51

experimental trends in medicine." Despite this favorable climate, there was a down side. The Church did not suddenly relinquish its great power, especially in Spain, where any theory that seemed possibly contrary to the scriptures or church doctrine was regarded with deep suspicion. Nevertheless, the period as a whole was one of great progress.

In order for there to be any real advance in contraceptive knowledge, it was necessary that there first be some understanding of the reproductive cycle in the female and the role of both the ovum and the sperm in the conception process. Discussion of this developing understanding will be followed by considerations of events leading to new birth control practices.

THE MICROSCOPE

Before the development of the microscope, there was only limited understanding of reproduction. Even after the instrument had become available to scientists, many questions remained unanswered.

Some historians credit Zacharias Janssen (1590), a Dutch maker of optical lenses, as the first to make a usable microscope. The great Galileo devised one in 1610 but he did not exploit his new invention, possibly because of his problems with the Inquisition. Others who worked with various magnifying instruments were A. B. Amici, Marcello Malpighi, Jan Swammerdam, Robert Hooke and Sir Isaac Newton (1642–1727).

Newton's microscope was of insufficient quality to make a significant contribution. Perhaps the great scientist did not appreciate its potential because his was a cosmic rather than microcosmic view. Matters that concerned him most were the law of gravitation, the motion of the planets and fluid mechanics. He must have felt that he could put lenses to better use in the telescope.

The name most usually associated with the origin of the science of microscopy is Antoni van Leeuwenhoek. Born in 1632, records indicate that van Leeuwenhoek's parents were respectable, but not of the aristocracy. His education was adequate but did not include the classics. On the other hand his favorite subject was mathematics, and in this field he excelled. Following completion of his studies he was apprenticed to a cloth merchant, and it was his interest in fabrics that led him to devise lenses in order to study the quality of a material and the weaving. The clear vision thus afforded led him to recognition of the scientific potential of these lenses, and what started as a hobby became a serious scientific pursuit. By 1671 his scientific career had begun. A wide-ranging interest in nature led him to examine hundreds of commonplace items through his magnifying instruments, which he constantly strove to improve. By the end of his career he had ground over 500 lenses and the best possessed a magnifying power of 270 together with a resolving power of 1.4 microns.

Leeuwenhoek's study of natural objects was fresh and unfettered by prevailing biological thought. This was so because he was unable to read Latin and he was therefore not exposed to some of the fashionable non-scientific belief then current. In this way his limited education brought the benefit of unbiased inquiry. He was influenced by writers in Dutch such as Cornelis Bontekoes on medicine and Swammerdam on insects. Not available to him were Hooke on microscopy, Grew on plant pathology and Redi on insects because he could not translate them, but he did learn from their illustrations.

Probably his most important discovery occurred in 1674 when his student Hamm first saw human spermatozoa. This was a giant step in the understanding of reproductive physiology. In 1677 Leeuwenhoek gave his account of this observation:

> 'I have diverse times examined the same matter (human semen) from a healthy man (not from a sick man nor spoiled by keeping for a long time, and not liquified after the lapse of some minutes, but immediately after ejaculation, before six beats of the pulse had intervened) and I have seen so great a number of living creatures in it, that sometimes more than a thousand were moving about in an amount of material the size of a grain of sand.
>
> These animacules were smaller than the corpuscles which impart a red color to the blood; so that I judge a million of them not equal in size to a large grain of sand. Their bodies were rounded, but blunt in front and running to a point behind, and transparent, and with the thickness of about one twenty-fifth that of the body; so that I can best liken them in form to a small earth nut with a long tail. The animacules moved forward with a snake-like motion of the tail, as eels do when swimming in water.'
>
> What I describe here was not obtained by any sinful contrivance on my part, but the observations were made upon the excess with which nature provided me in my conjugal relations.'

Despite this later disclaimer, Leeuwenhoek was severely criticized in some quarters.

It is clear that he did not completely understand the female contribution to conception, largely because the human egg had not yet been identified. His friend, de Graaf, had described the ovarian follicle which bears his name, and Leeuwenhoek went as far as to realize that the follicle was too large to pass down the Fallopian tube. Since the understanding of the ovulation

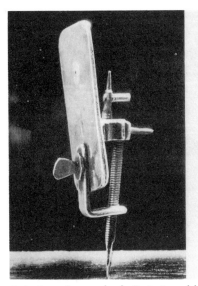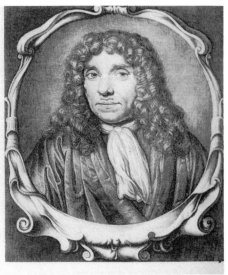

Antoni van Leeuwenhoek. Portrait, and his microscope. (Courtesy of Museum Boerhaave, Leiden)

process was incomplete, work with the microscope gave birth to two incompatable explanations concerning conception. Niklass Hartsoeker (1650–1725) wrote in 1684 his essay, "Essai de Dioptrique" that he could identify a pre-formed human within the sperm. Those who accepted his observations were convinced that the male only was responsible for new life (the Animaculists) and that the female served only as an incubator. Others considered the female as the major contributor (the Ovists). The later champion of the latter theory was Spallanzani.

AFTER LEEUWENHOEK

There was no consensus concerning the theories of generation even after Leeuwenhoek and Hamm described the human spermatozoa. It is characteristic of the confused situation that Drelincourt, in 1685, suggested the Graafian follicle contained the ovum. This notion has been described by Professor Victor Medvei as "a cry in the wilderness." The scientific community was sharply divided, not only between Ovists and Animaculists, but there were also those who believed in spontaneous generation, even in animals and humans. This idea came from the observation that some creatures seemed to develop *de novo*; maggots develop "spontaneously" in offal. Relatedly, many believed that virgin birth was possible quite apart from divine intervention.

It seems strange today that the importance of the egg was discounted by so many scientists. In the avian order its significance was certainly understood. There was a well known Latin phrase, *"Omne vivum ex ovo"* — "All life comes from the egg." Even before the Christian era, the egg symbolized birth, life and resurrection as evidenced in ancient Egypt where it was customary to place eggs in tombs. Later, of course, in Christian times, the egg became a part of Easter symbolism. The Ovists believed in the supremacy of the egg. William Harvey (1578–1637) wrote in *De Generatione* that the egg was the source of all life. Some of the ancients clearly recognized that both male and female elements were important. The early Hindus believed that the semen combined with menstrual blood to produce conception, and the Egyptians also had an understanding, as shown in a hymn composed to the sun god Aton by Amenophis IV:

> "Creator of the germ in woman
> Maker of the seed in man
> Giving life to the son
> In the body of the mother."

Yet in the seventeenth century the role of the egg was still frequently dismissed.

Compte George Louis Buffon (1707–1788) set out to cover all scientific knowledge in his 44 volume *Histoire Naturelle*. One of his chief interests was in the process of generation. He did not believe in the animality of sperm, considering semen to be mere aggregation of organic matter. When John Needham, an English Catholic priest, moved to Paris, he and Buffon decided to work together. Their skills were complementary, Needham being an expert microscopist and Buffon an outstanding theorist. The latter postulated that the ejaculate contained molecules which were indestructible and undefinable, which nature used again and again to form new organisms. He concluded that this material, in the proper environment (*"moule interieur"*) could form new organisms (thus, spontaneous generation). Needham and Buffon were most likely ignorant of the experiments reported by Francisco Redi in 1668 (*Esperienze intorno alla generazione degli insetti*). The gifted Redi, a celebrated author and poet, outlined in unrivaled prose his classical experiments disproving that animals could arise *de novo*. Unaware of this work, Needham and Buffon performed experiments designed to prove the theory of spontaneous generation. Micro-organisms were placed in flasks and then killed by heat. The flasks, which had been sealed with mastic, were not airtight so airborne bacteria soon recolonized the containers.

The next actor in this scientific drama was Lazzaro Spallanzani (1729–1799). Professor Victor Medvei characterized him as the possessor of one of the most versatile minds of his time. He had started his career as a lawyer but when that profession failed to offer sufficient challenge he turned to science. Spallanzani became professor of logic and metaphysics, first at Reggio, then Modena and finally at Pavia. High on his agenda was an effort to disprove the theory of spontaneous generation which he considered senseless. His experiments were similar to those of Needham and Buffon except that his flasks were sealed hermetically by flaming. No organisms subsequently grew in his airtight flasks. His report led to a scientific duel between himself and Needham and Buffon, a dispute characterized by lost tempers, deviousness and unseemly vituperation.

Traditionally the clergy, the medical profession and scientists have been held to be honest and charitable (the various depictions of the Mad Scientist to the contrary notwithstanding). Unfortunately, in reality, controversy has always been part of the scientific scene. Overt fraud occasionally occurs — a modern instance is depicted in *The Patchwork Mouse* by J. Hixon. Even disagreements among palentologists and between them and molecular biologists concerning identification and aging of ancient hominids are not always conducted with kid gloves. A recent book, *Bones of Contention* by R. Lewin details some errant behavior.

Spallanzani also demonstrated that fertilization could not take place in the absence of semen. He covered the male part of the frog with linen and observed that conception did not occur after mating. Further, Spallanzani was able to fertilize frog ova that had been placed on filter paper. This work refuted the dictum of Linnaeus who had said, "never, in any living body, does fecundation or impregnantion take place outside the body of the mother."

Curiously, Spellanzani thought that the fluid of the semen was the active principal, even in the absence of sperm. This had led many to consider him an Ovist or one who believes that the egg contains the elements of a new individual and that the semen only provides nourishment in some way. In a complete analysis of the question Medvei points out that Spallanzani did not tailor his experiments to prove a theory of preformation. In retrospect, it is clear that in his experiments he used seminal fluid thought to be free of sperm, but which did, in fact, contain spermatozoa.

Despite this scientist's convincing work, the theory of spontaneous generation was still believed by some until the great Louis Pasteur, one hundred years later, repeated the experiments showing that sterile, airtight flasks remained free of micro-organisms. Only then was the entire scientific community convinced.

Other milestones in the development of knowledge of reproductive physiology were the report, 42 years after Spallanzani, by Rudolph von Koelleker that sperm originated in the testes, and the discovery in 1827 of the mammalian ovum by Carl Ernst von Baer. He published his finding in his work, *De Ovi Mammalium et Hominis Genesi*. It is interesting that Drelincourt, back in 1685, had suggested that the ovum might be contained within the Graafian follicle; his suggestion, however, received no scientific attention.

The discovery of the mammalian ovum in 1827 by Carl Ernst von Baer, was a great step toward the eventual elucidation of the human reproductive process. Spermatozoa had previously been discovered, as we have noted, by Leeuwenhoek and his student Hamm. In 1865 Franz Schweiger-Seidel showed that the individual sperm cell possessed both a nucleus and cytoplasm. The first observation of the union of sperm and ovum was made by Martin Barry in 1843. Oscar Hertwig then, in 1875, observed that the sperm actually entered the ovum. The conclusion could then be drawn that the resulting organism contained the genetic properties of both parents. It was later discovered (1883) by Edouard van Beneden that each germ cell had reduced its chromosome count by one half. The fertilized ovum was thus equipped with a full compliment of genetic material. Huxley later poetically characterized the process, "the warp was derived from the female and the woof from the male".

The idea that there existed an internal chemical control over reproduction (as well as other body functions) was first suggested by Theophile de Bordeu in 1775. His talent was in theory rather than experimentation so proof was lacking. He believed that the body economy was dependent on certain substances that were passed into the circulatory system and which then acted on targeted organs. He was particularly interested in "maleness" or "femaleness" and specifically identified both the ovary and testes as organs that imparted "tone to all parts". He observed that eunuchs possessed physical and behavioral characteristics that differed from the normal (unspayed). Bordeu has the best claim to be considered the father of modern endocrinology. His successor at Montpelier introduced the term "vital principle" (*vitatis agens*) to denote internal secretions which in turn caused an "hormonic equilibrium".

It is clear that a complete understanding of reproductive physiology was necessary in order to develop sound methods of birth control. Some scientists far too early believed that everything there was to know was already known. Before Columbus discovered the New World, the escutcheon of the Spanish royal family contained representations of the Pillars of Hercules (the Straits of Gibraltar in Europe and the Jebel Musa in Africa), with the motto, "*Ne plus ultra*" — there is nothing beyond. Later the "*ne*" had to be dropped, for there was more beyond. So it was with the science of reproductive physiology, which did not appear full grown like Athena from the head of Zeus.

The spontaneous generation imbroglio was not an event unique in science, past or present. Doctor D. G. Wilson, writing in the Journal of the Royal Society of Medicine, says that, "Physicians yearn for the precision of science but sit amongst the mess and fuzz of humanity." Deeply embedded ideas are hard to abandon. He says further that it appears to be more difficult to discard a learned false theory than to learn a new one. This is a problem with which doctors have always had to contend, and scientists can effectively back themselves into a corner by being unwilling to unlearn. As the psalmist said, "He has made a pit and digged it, And is fallen into the ditch which he made". Mistakes are part of discovery and even today scientists go astray by tending to retain established hypotheses even when new discoveries are failing to support them. Scientific inquiry can consequently become very unscientific.

ORGASM AND CONCEPTION

It was apparent, even to the ancients, that male orgasm was necessary for ejaculation and therefore for conception. On the other hand female orgasm was not as well understood. Some thought that it tended to increase fertility and others that it decreased the likelihood of conception. Most biologists now believe that it is a phenomenon seen only in humans. Sexual physiologists theorize that it is related to the typical face to face position which allows for more intimate contact through verbal and tactile stimuli.

The role of female orgasm has been debated since ancient times. Soranus, the greatest gynecologist of antiquity, believed that passionate intercourse tended to cause fruitfulness. Ismail Jurjani: addressed the question in his

Treasures of Medicine (c. AD 1110). His view was that simultaneous orgasm should be avoided unless pregnancy was desired.

The early Christian teaching, based on the philosophy of St Paul, was that sex was sinful. He even opposed marriage, but said "it is better to marry than to burn". Even though male orgasm was necessary it was allowed only if one hated it. Active participation by the female was discouraged. Reproduction was the only reason for sexual congress, and mutual enjoyment was thought to cause sterility and was evil. Female orgasm was therefore considered bad.

Confusion concerning the role of female orgasm in reproduction persisted until modern times. The issue was addressed in 1709 by R. D. Carolus Musitanus in his book *Women's Diseases*.

> "Passionate coitus is to be avoided for it is unfruitful. Sometimes the woman does not draw back her buttocks (as Soranus directs) and conquers, as is the custom of Spanish women, who move their whole bodies while they have intercourse from an excess of voluptuousness (they are extraordinarily passionate) and perform the Phygian dance and some passionately sing a song, which in Spanish is called *chaccara*, and on account of this (sic) Spanish women are sterile".

Most Victorian physiologists thought that female passiveness decreased the likelihood of conception — an idea not borne out by the large size of most families during that period of female repression.

It is now recognized that female orgasm is not necessary for conception. However, its importance in marital harmony is certain. The woman should not be merely a sexual object whose function is only for the satisfaction of male libido. Coitus is a form of human communication that involves both parties and should be mutually rewarding.

5

Population Science

PRE-MALTHUSIAN ATTITUDES TO POPULATION CONTROL

Over-population has been a concern of mankind since the dawn of civilization. When natural disasters or those made by man failed to keep human population density at the beneficial level, some sort of reproductive restriction was clearly needed. Since contraceptive practices have been necessary at times throughout history, many of the world's most influential thinkers and writers have had occasion to discuss it.

Imaginative writers have often dramatized human suffering, some of it attributable to over-population factors. In the preface to *Les Misérables*, Victor Hugo wrote:

> "So long as there shall exist, by reason of law and custom, a social condemnation, which in the face of civilization artificially creates hell on earth and complicates a destiny that is divine with human fatality, so long as the three problems of that age — the degradation of man by poverty, the ruin of women by starvation and the dwarfing of childhood by physical and spiritual blight — are not solved: so long as in certain religions social asphixia shall be possible in other words, and from yet a more extended point of view, so long as ignorance and misery remain on earth, books like this cannot be needless".

Although Hugo did not specifically mention birth control, what other social condemnation and social asphyxia could he have meant? Starvation and female misery are caused by several circumstances but certainly unrestricted reproduction is one. Perhaps Hugo was somewhat responsible for the French acceptance of population control. Colin Clark in "World Population" (*Nature*, 1958) said that Britain did not listen to Malthus but France did.

Both Plato and Aristotle warned of the dangers of over-population. Tertullian (Quintus Septimus Floren Tertullianus) was one of the most influential early Christian writers; he was also a significant and uncannily prophetic commentator on the problem of over-population. Born in AD 155 to a father who was a pro-consul in Carthage, he studied law and progressed to become an eminent jurist. The circumstances which caused his conversion to Christianity are not known, but as a Christian he sought to unite primitive Christian belief with intellectual consistency and interpretation. He addressed the problem of over-population in *De Anima*, one of his many writings, commenting on the blessings of catastrophes. He noted that "the strongest witness is the vast population of the earth to which we are a burden and she scarcely can provide for our needs; as our demands grow greater, our complaints against nature's inadequacy are heard by all. The scourges of pestilence, famine, wars, and earthquakes have come to be regarded as a blessing to overcrowded nations, since they prune away the luxuriant growth of the human race". The desperation of tone in this quote sounds surprisingly modern, but since he was an advocate of the teachings of the New Testament, it seems highly unlikely that he seriously supported any theory that disasters were beneficial to mankind. At the time he wrote *De Anima* he was a follower of Montamus, who claimed powers of prophecy, and perhaps this accounts for the seer-like authority of his utterance.

Polybius (c. 280 BC), a Greek historian of the School of Thucydides, offers a contrary view. While he is said personally to have lacked grace, this is not apparent in the five surviving of his 40 books. Polybius' thoughts were most likely influenced by his experiences and travels. Following the defeat of Perseus of Macedonia he was deported to Rome where his talent was recognized by one of his captors, the great Roman General Scipio. While serving as aide to the general he witnessed the great destruction and loss of life and property at Carthage and Corinth. These events made him fear for the further growth of mankind; depopulation seemed the threat. It must be added that his views were always expressed in a dispassionate manner because he loathed exaggeration. His theory was that "a historian should not try to astonish his readers".

Moving to the period of the English Renaissance, Sir Thomas More realized that there could not be an ideal community without some form of population control. He advised in *Utopia*,

> "That the city neither be depopulated nor grow beyond measure, provision is made that no household shall have fewer than ten or more than sixteen adults; there are six thousand such households in each city, apart from its surrounding territory. Of children under age, of course, no number can be fixed. This limit is easily observed by transferring those who exceed the number in larger families into those that are

under the prescribed number. Whenever all the families of a city reach
their full quota, the adults in excess of that number help to make up
the deficient population of other cities".

Of course, the concern here is more with population deployment (for optimal
social structure) than with population limitation. In contrast, Martin Luther
was, at about the same time, attributing responsibility for population size
entirely to God. He said "*Gott dacht Kinder, der wir sie euch ernaheren*".

Queen Elizabeth I clearly recognised the problem caused by crowding.
In the 31st year of her reign she had a statute passed which provided that
every cottage must have at least four acres of land permanently attached.
Unfortunately, this law did not remain in force after her death. In the
Elizabethan period, as in most times when there is a low literacy level,
custom governs behavior strongly, including attitudes towards family size.
Economic pressure (poverty or the perceived proximity of it) frequently
induces a high birth rate. Sir Francis Bacon (1561–1626) was well aware of
the power of custom and how the ability to look ahead thoughtfully was
rare. He commented: "Satisfaction with the present induces neglect of the
future". In another essay he considers the effort and responsibility associated
with reproduction: "He that hath wife and children hath given hostages to
fortune". (Patriarchial authority is clearly suggested, too).

When European countries became overcrowded, emigration to the colonies
became popular. Robert Burton noted in his *The Anatomy of Melancholy*
(1621) that, "if people overbound they shall be eased by colonies". Action
needs to be taken at home too, in Burton's opinion; it is not enough to rely
on the safety-valve effect of the colonies. He advises that appropriate policy
would be for the number of children per couple to be controlled by men
not marrying before the age of 25 and women not before 20 years of age.

Jonathan Swift (1667–1745) was an acute observer of the problems of
the human race, and during his years as Dean of the Cathedral of St. Patrick's
in Dublin, he was stirred to produce several satires commenting on social
ills. He noted that there are few nations where at least one-third of the
population is not deprived of some of the necessities of life.

Swift had no coherent social policy but was, according to the critic
Kathleen Williams, convinced that proper Christian behavior was the only
answer to the "chaos of human motives". Swift's dark outlook perceived
man as not at all naturally good but dominated by self love, faltering reason
and disruptive passions. In his shocking essay "A Modest Proposal for
Preventing the Children of Ireland from Being a Burden to Their Parents or
Country" he alludes to the contemporary problems in Ireland of oppression,

poverty and excess population. He says, in the introduction, "It is a melancholy object to those who walk through this great town (Dublin) or travel in the country when they see the streets, the roads and cabin doors crowded with beggars of the female sex, followed by three, four or six children, all in rags, and importuning every passenger for an alms". Swift goes on, with outward logic but terrifying irony, to suggest that an all-round solution will be achieved if the babies of the Irish poor are eaten ("boiled, roast or as a fricasseé") by the wealthy English. His attitude combines perception of out-of-control population growth with fury over English oppression.

Benjamin Franklin (1706–1750) was one of the most original thinkers of his time and had an attitude towards population growth which reflected his standpoint as representative of a new nation anxious to grow in strength and take full possession of the "new" continent. Population growth, a natural force, is seen as regulated by the availability of "subsistence" and vital in its creation of new political realities. In 1755 he wrote,

> "There is no bounds to the prolific nature of plants or animals, but what is made by their crowding and interfering with each other's means of subsistence — in fine, a nation, well regulated, is like a polypus: take away a limb, its place is soon supplied, cut it in two, and each deficient part shall speedily grow out of the remaining. Thus if you have room for subsistence enough, as you may, by dividing ten polypuses out of one, you may of one make ten nations equally populous and powerful; or rather increase the nation tenfold in numbers and strength".

The analogy that Franklin used to illustrate the rapid growth of human populations was that of the reproductive process of lower animals, i.e. one individual divides into two (parthenogenetic or asexual reproduction). To further his thought, Franklin noted that from an estimated 80,000 early British immigrants there were, by 1755, over one million descendants.

Thomas Malthus was reputedly influenced by Franklin's observation in 1755 on population growth (Malthus' first essay was written in 1783). Since many before him voiced concern about over-population, why is Malthus special? Sir William Osler said, "In science it is not the first that makes the observation that deserves the credit; rather it should go to the one who convinces the world". Similarly the philosopher Alfred North Whitehead observed, "We give credit not to the first man who has an idea but to the first one to take it seriously". It would be an exaggeration to say that Malthus convinced the world, but he more than anyone before him brought the problem of population control to the attention of many thinking people.

MALTHUS AND THE SCIENTIFIC CLIMATE OF THE EARLY 19TH CENTURY

According to Will and Ariel Durant, in England in the 19th Century the shift, begun in the 18th Century, from a basically agricultural economy to an industrialized one, accelerated. Understanding of this great change was underpinned to a considerable extent by development in mathematics. Although England surrendered leadership in mathematics to the French, it was mathematics that Malthus used to support his theories. Malthus' work and its implications seem to prefigure H. G. Wells' viewpoint articulated many years later: "Statistical thinking will one day be as necessary for efficient citizenship as the ability to read and write".

Malthus was almost the first social scientist to apply statistics to the analysis of population growth. This combination of methods was to become the science of demography, a term first used in 1880. Lord Kelvin made the point about statistics unequivocally: "When you can measure what you are speaking about, you know something about it; but when you cannot express it in numbers — you have scarcely advanced to the stage of science". Since Malthus' time, analysts have modified his mathematical formula for working, but most consider it basically sound.

Thomas Robert Malthus was born near Guildford, Surrey, on February 13, 1766. He was the sixth of seven children born to Henrietta and Daniel Malthus. His father was a prosperous and intellectual man who numbered among his friends many of the scholars of his day, including David Hume. He was an ardent admirer of Jean Jacques Rousseau, and it was the latter's book, *Emile*, that provided the source of his ideas concerning education. Home life was characterized by lively and stimulating conversations. Young Thomas, called Robert by family and friends, received his early education at home. Later he was sent first to study under Richard Graves at Claverton and then to the Dissenting Academy where his professor was Gilbert Wakefield. Thomas showed an early interest in mathematics and soon became intrigued by data analysis. Concerning the reliance on mathematics, James Clerk Maxwell (1831–1879) a hundred years later wrote: "There is nothing more essential to the right understanding of things than a perception of the relations of number".

Malthus finished his education in 1788 and received his Master of Arts degree in 1791. He made friends easily and enjoyed an active social life, seeming not in the least inhibited by a birth defect of a cleft palate and a hare lip. His was a generally analytical mind, one that liked to examine both

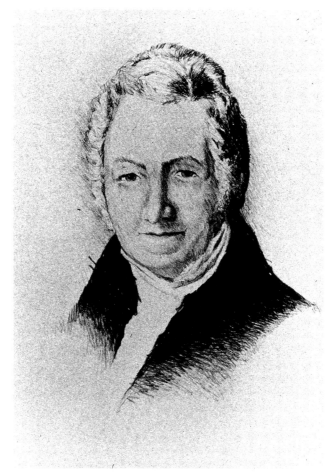

Thomas Malthus. (Drawing by artist Scott Fuller, from a portrait by J. Linnell, 1833)

sides of any question. For example, he described the French Revolution as a "blazing comet destined either to inspire with fresh life or scorch up and destroy". During his college days, his best friend was William Otter, later Bishop of Chichester. Following completion of his studies, he was ordained in the Anglican Church and became curate at Okewood in Surrey. In 1793 he was elected a fellow of Jesus College, a position he held until his marriage to Harriet Eckersall in 1804. The following year he became professor of history and political economy at the East India Company's College at Haileybury. This was the first academic post ever offered in political science. He was elected to membership in the Royal Society of London and was one of the founders of the Statistical Society of London in 1834. Foreign recognition came when he was elected to the French Académie des Sciences and the Royal Academy of Berlin.

During his later years Malthus remained intellectually active, writing essays on political economy. He died in December, 1834, and was buried in the Abbey Church at Bath

MALTHUS ON PROBLEMS OF POPULATION AND POVERTY

When Malthus began to ponder about the relationship between population and subsistence he could perceive problems. It worried him that some of the thinkers of the time were not intellectually honest and that others prostituted their understanding to their self-interest (as members of a certain class); in such a situation truth suffered. He pointed out that traditional study of history was of little help because it was written by and about the upper classes and did not include evaluation of the lives of the poor. The conviction grew in him that the unequal ratio between population and the means of subsistence commonly brought about consequences similar to those of the barbarian invasions and where peasants were killed and productive land ruined.

Malthus and his father had many debates about Godwin's book, *Enquiry Concerning Political Justice* (1793). Young Malthus was critical of this as no more than Utopian fantasy. He pointed out that its philosophy was inconsistent with the Book of Ecclesiastes which proclaimed that when food was in excess an increase in population followed. Malthus added that, if population continues to increase, a point will be reached where the earth's agriculture will be unable to supply enough food for all.

Malthus' first essay, "On the Principal of Population" was published anonymously in 1798 and his last appeared in 1805. All but the first were signed by him and there seems to have been little doubt concerning the authorship of the first. His conclusions were clearly stated: "Assuming, then, my postulata as granted, I say that the power of population is infinitely greater than the power in the earth to produce subsistence for man. Population when unchecked increases in a geometrical ratio, subsistence only in an arithmetical ratio. A slight acquaintance with number will show the immensity of the first power in comparison to the second". (The ratio for human increase is 1−2−4−8−16, etc., that for subsistence is 1−2−3−4−5, etc.) "That population cannot increase without the means of subsistence is a proposition so evident that it needs no illustration". He further stated that "to remedy the frequent distresses of the common people, the Poor Laws of England have been instituted; but it is to be feared that although they may have alleviated a little the intensity of individual misfortune, they have spread the general evil over a much larger surface". In short, Malthus' position is that when subsistence is available, population increases to take it up. Population is effectively restricted (if at the cost of human suffering) by the unavailability of subsistence. "Indulgence" of the poor beyond their capacity to contribute to increased output (and therefore greater subsistence) is policy leading to increased population and so a worsened situation. Malthus' solution to the population problem was delayed marriage and strict pre-marital chastity, and he called this "moral restraint".

Malthus' views were attacked on several grounds. Those who believed in the perfectability of man, i.e., Godwin and the elder Malthus, and the followers of Rousseau, considered his views unacceptably pessimistic. Some persons considered Malthus' lack of sympathy for the poor unforgivable. According to Ardrey, Malthus' apparent disregard for the plight of the poor (he even advocated the abolition of parish charity) offended the religious convictions of the time. Condorcet was similarly sympathetic toward the poor and envisioned a Welfare State. He said, "All social institutions should have for their aim the physical, intellectual and moral betterment of the most numerous and poorest class". He had anticipated Malthus' theory but advocated birth control rather than "moral restraint".

However those who shared Rousseau's anti-clerical bias would not be inclined to support the views of a curate. Many of the philosophers and social scientists of Malthus' time shared this bias. Part of their rejection of Malthus' theories was because he was a curate of the episcopal church. Foremost among the dissidents was Jean Jacques Rousseau. To clarify Rousseau's views it must be stated that he had advised that marriage be entered into only after careful consideration. He further advised that sexual congress be infrequent. Whether the population problem influenced his thinking in this subject is conjectural. Rousseau also advocated early and careful sexual education in the belief that it would encourage moral behavior. He also felt that every individual should have the right to express his or her own will but that the common needs of the community must be considered.

Others of Malthus' detractors doubted that population density would ever surpass the food supply. Most critics thought it inconceivable that population growth could ever be controlled by delayed marriage, strict pre-marital chastity and "moral restraint".

The publication of Malthus' essays may have astonished the critics but it certainly did not render them speechless. Godwin, Coleridge and Hazlitt attacked Malthus' theories in a manner that seemed "outside the limits of academic brawling"; Carlisle called them "The Dismal Science". Malthus took the criticisms with good grace and seemed to accept them as a cross he had inevitably to bear.

On the other hand, William Pitt the Younger withdrew his Poor Law bill after reading one of the essays. Malthus had pointed out that this law would only intensify suffering in the long run. The brilliant economist, David Ricardo, became an ardent supporter, and both Alfred Russell Wallace and Charles Darwin stated that Malthus' work influenced them in the development of the theory of natural selection. Perhaps they were impressed by Malthus' observation quite possibly humorous that when the genes of a member of an ancient fictional family, the Bickerstaffs, were crossed with those of Maud, a milkmaid, the complexion and height of their offspring were improved.

> "The capacity of improvement in plants and animals, to a certain degree, no person can possibly doubt.
>
> It does not, by any means, seem impossible that by intention to breed, a certain degree of improvement, similar to that among animals, might take place among men.
>
> I know of no well-directed attempts of this kind except in the ancient family of the Bickerstaffs, who are said to have been very successful in whitening the skin and increasing the height of their race by prudent marriages, particularly by that very judicious cross with Maud, the milkmaid, by which some capital defects in the constitution of the family were corrected".

In general, although there were those who sought to suppress the essays, the British custom of free speech neutralized this tendency.

Malthus' ideas were no doubt influenced by conditions in England of the time. Early marriage was encouraged; girls could marry at 12 and boys at 14. Bordellos, both hetero- and homosexual, were common. Divorce was rare and expensive and could only be obtained by an act of Parliament.

The birth control movement can be considered a direct result of Malthus' theories and writings. The more practical minded social reformers came to regard his methods of population control, i.e., later marriage, strict pre-marital chastity and "moral restraint", as not acceptable to most of the population, and that other methods were needed. It was this search of the Neo-Malthusians for more practical methods which led to the achievements of Francis Place, Jeremy Bentham and others.

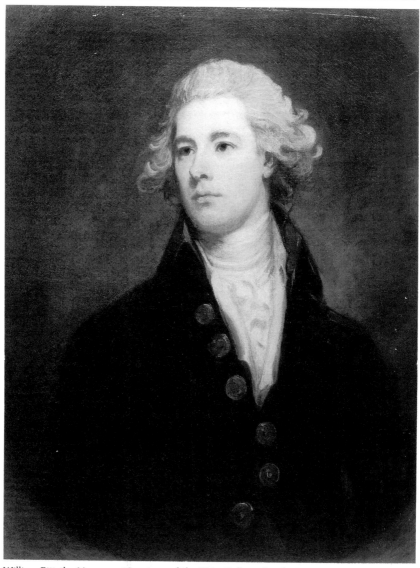

William Pitt the Younger. (Courtesy of the Tate Gallery, London)

The contribution of Bentham was considerable. A social reformer and founder of the Utilitarian movement, he was also the first to advocate a contraceptive in the form of a vaginal sponge; this he did one year before Malthus' essay. He also proposed a registry for population statistics — clearly a recommendation owing something to Malthus.

AFTER MALTHUS

The judgment of posterity must be that Malthus had great insight and an effective passion to prove his thesis. He seems to have recognised that there was stagnation of beliefs among the ruling classes, and he had the graciousness to accept resistance and ideas contrary to his, while trying to engender a new philosophy. All human knowledge falls short of absolute truth and Hume said that even mathematical science is only approximate truth. Nevertheless, Malthus' theory has stood the test of time well. His prescribed solutions, however, have not, because the only real solution to population problems is birth control and this Thomas Malthus would never have accepted.

Indeed it was only in the later editions of his writings that he stressed his characteristic solution of "moral restraint", i.e. postponement of marriage, strict pre-marital chastity and avoidance of vice. That this advocacy of "moral restraint" was *not* practical would certainly have occurred to Malthus, considering his knowledge of sexuality, and it seems he remained pessimistic concerning any effective curbs on sexual passions.

Despite the lack of equivalence between the solutions endorsed by Malthus (who did not endorse any type of artificial contraception) and those suggested by the early birth control advocates, the latter were dubbed Neo-Malthusians. These Neo-Malthusians were not physicians — professional medical men were not part of early efforts to promote birth control. Professor Himes has noted that, in general, society frowned on doctors who supported the movement. Those far-sighted ones who were the exception and did support family planning were perceived as returning to the classical attitude. As Professor Himes notes, "In antiquity anti-conceptional technique had a definite place in preventive medicine", and physicians exposed to public question because of their acceptance of birth control needs were glad to make use of classical precedent.

One of the assumed benefits of population control was that it might blunt the instinctive drive to possess territory. Many armed conflicts have been started because of the need of more room for an increasing population. The German concept of *Lebensraum* is considered by historians to have been a major factor in causing both World Wars. In corroboration, animal studies have shown increasing aggressiveness when conditions are crowded. Social studies on both man and animals have shown that both instinctively require an area of inviolable space surrounding the individual or tribe. This "territorial imperative" has been described by Robert Ardrey in *The Social Contract*, but it is important to be aware that both men and animals do demonstrate that adaptive behavior is possible. Japanese society exhibits stratification features and customs that contribute to acceptable behavior under conditions of very high population density.

WAS MALTHUS RIGHT? SOME LATER APPRAISALS

John Stuart Mill (1806–1873) shared Malthus' views concerning population: "Even in a progressive state of capital, in old countries, a conscientious or prudential restraint on population is indispensible to prevent the increase of numbers from outstripping the increase in capital, and the condition of the classes who are at the bottom of society from being deteriorated". Mill clearly felt for the poor and advocated reproductive restraint. His failure to define the *modus operandi* was possibly due to his sense of delicacy concerning sexual matters, what he termed "delicate sentiments of virtue". His thinking was no doubt influenced by that of his father, James Mill, a contemporary of Malthus and a close friend of Jeremy Bentham.

In 1922 Sir Alexander Carr-Saunders vehemently denounced Malthus' views in his book, *The Population Problem*. However, Harvard Professor E.O. Wilson reasoned that competition occurs only when there is a severe shortage in an essential resource.

Robert Ardrey (writing in 1950) believed that Malthus was wrong. This belief was based on the premise that before population came to outgrow the food supply, effective correcting factors such as birth control would be adopted. He went so far as to advise that contraception should be encouraged by placing taxation on families with "surplus" children. Other factors such as economic advantages for bachelors and spinsters were advocated, and he also suggested that abortion be made legal; measures such as these have been adopted by China. Ardrey further suggested that foreign aid be withheld from countries which made no effort to control population.

Many modern writers have developed the conviction that over-population is the major problem in parts of the world. A. L. Cochrane in 1972 argued that this was the case in England. He added that to convince the public of this fact was difficult.

Following the French Revolution and up to World War II there was, in fact, a decline in population growth in Western Europe. John Hajnal in an essay in 1968 noted that if one drew a line from Trieste to Leningrad, the "nuptiality patterns" differed from one side of the line to the other. In the west, the proportion of married women aged 15 to those aged 50 was no more than 45% to 50%, whereas east of the line and in Africa and Asia, the proportion was 60% to 70%. In addition, natural birth control measures were taken by many women in the western area. These included late marriage, prolonged lactation and abstinence. Coitus interruptus was widely practised. In Western Europe the decrease in the marital fertility was of the order of 50% or more, compared to the Eastern European countries.

The situation in the United States is similar to that west of Hajnal's line. In 1800 American white women were having more children than their Western European counterparts, but this trend had reversed by 1900. The average American woman in 1800 had an average of 7.04 children; by 1900 the figure had dropped to 3.56.

Thus, the decrease in population growth in the west together with the increase in productivity occasioned by the Industrial Revolution made Malthus' theories seem obsolete to many.

This assessment was not shared by Professor Arnold Toynbee, who addressed the population problem in his short book, *An Historian's Approach to Religion* (1956) having unaccountably neglected to discuss it in his 12-volume *History of the World*. Toynbee wrote:

> "A change in social habits is required to lower the birth rate and this is an affair of the heart; and even in an advanced and progressively minded country the heart cannot easily be moved to go faster than its habitually slow gait. The time lag of 140 years in Britain between the head's effect and the heart's effect upon the movement of population is unlikely to have been longer than the average, and during the interval the population of Britain increased nearly fourfold".
>
> "It could hardly be hoped that the change of social habits necessary for stabilizing the world's population through a voluntary reduction of the birth rate could be achieved before the increase in the world's population would reach the limit of the number that could be fed, even if the world's food production were to have been raised to the highest degree that could be achieved by the systematic application of science. In that event, Malthus's forecast would have been wrong only in antedating the crisis by a mere 100 years or thereabouts and the inevitable consequence would be a further restriction on freedom — and this time in a field in which governmental interference had been almost unheard of hitherto".

In another work, *Reconsiderations: A Study of History* (1961) Toynbee wrote:

> "In a society in which public hygiene has been achieving sensational progressive reduction in the death rate, a reduction in the birth rate on a corresponding scale is required if technology's potential gift of a higher standard of living, spiritual as well as material, is not to be

swallowed up by a sensational increase in the number of mouths to be fed.

Hitherto, the majority of mankind has, as a matter of course, always multipled and replenished the earth up to the limits allowed by its food supply at a subsistence level only just above the starvation line; unless this habit is abandoned, modern technology will have brought with it, for the majority, no decrease in miserable numbers".

So at the last Arnold Toynbee analyses Malthus' theory and its ultimate effect on civilization. This is important since Toynbee's life work has been to study the history of man and from that to make some conclusions as to where we have been and what predictions can be made from past events. As we can see he counsels reproductive restraint. No longer can we depend on the sovereignty of ancient gods. Clearly human action is needed or else the "enterprise of civilization" is doomed. Toynbee's hope is that man's history will not appear exclusively a matter of chaos or chance. There has to be some order and pattern and a partially predictable regularity in human behavior.

POPULATION CONTROL AND GENETIC QUALITY

Robert Cook in 1951 addressed the controversial problem of possible genetic deterioration. This possibility has occurred to many in the past. Homer had Nestor say to Telemachus, "Few men are equal to their fathers and for the most part lesser". That this is not always the case is clear. It does seem, however, that persons of exceptional ability tend to have fewer children than the average. Cook continues, saying the "plus genes" (favorable) do occur in the underprivileged; he terms this "cold storage reserve against the future". Some sociologists contend that, for reasons not clear, the intelligence of children born into large families is lower than that of the children of small families. Studies by Lorimer and Osborn in the United States and by Sir Godfrey Thompson in Scotland have confirmed this thesis. This does not, however, support any theory of defective genes, because nutrition, childhood illness and exposure to learning certainly influence an individual's I.Q. In his book *Human Fertility: The Modern Dilemma* (1971), Cook comes to the striking conclusion that the intelligentsia should act responsibly by increasing the size of their families. He feels that this is a necessary response to a world facing a genetic as well as a population crisis:

"A program of worldwide reorientation is important and must go hand in hand with dissemination of the new contraceptives. In the low birth countries, the spread of birth control among the more privileged has

established existing birth differentials which are now a serious threat
to future genetic quality".

In support of this radical policy, a program of "basic biological education"
is called for. Cook's view and recommendations constitute a crucial challenge
to the capacity of human nature to change; the outcome is uncertain, of
course.

6

The Birth Control Movement

The Industrial Revolution, beginning in the middle of the eighteenth century, resulted in dramatic changes in the world economy. The poor, no longer tied to the land, chose city life and industrial employment. What began as a dream became for many a nightmare. Social reformers in Europe, such philosophers as Hume, Rousseau and Condorcet, justices such as Sir John Holt and enlightened legislators such as William Pitt the Younger and clerics such as Thomas Malthus had anticipated the problems of poverty, crowding, over-population and health hazards. To these thinkers it was clear that some reform was necessary.

In America a similar situation existed. There was a vast migration from farms to cities and the problem was compounded by the large influx of immigrants. Poverty and misery existed in the New World as in the Old. It was clear that population control was an essential ingredient of meaningful reform, and thus the Birth Control Movement began on both sides of the Atlantic.

THE BIRTH CONTROL MOVEMENT IN BRITAIN

The movement got under way in the first part of the nineteenth century. The early innovators were hampered by the moral climate of the times. There was a strong contrast between publicly declared values and actual behavior. Modern scholarship has revealed by just how much middle-class Victorian values were underrepresentive of society as a whole. John Addington Symonds perceived this dualism and described it with unsympathetic abruptness: "Beneath the surface of brilliant social culture lurked gross appetites and savage passions, unrestrained by medieval piety, untutored by modern experience." The novels of Charles Dickens, with their linkage of gutter suffering to upper class hypocrisy, comprised one the the great voices of protest of the times. Many of those wishing to reduce the misery of the lower classes by, among other measures, introduction of realistic attitudes towards birth control, met blinkered outrage and sublimated guilt from those defending the ideals of the comfortable upper classes.

The laurel for *founder* of the Birth Control Movement in England is usually awarded to Francis Place (1771–1854). He was born into a large poverty-stricken family. His father was a brutal man characterized, Francis recorded, by behavior governed "almost wholly by his passions and animal sensations." Relief only came to the family when the elder Place disappeared for months at a time, but during these periods it fell to Place's mother to support the family by doing needlework. It is hard to resist the speculation that such a family background gave urgency and commitment to Place's later searching for means by which family life might be less pressed upon by "passions and animal sensations." He attributed his eventual success as a reformer more directly to the influence of two women other than his mother: one a schoolteacher who engendered in him a love of literature and books, and the other his wife whom he married in 1791 when he was 20.

By dint of hard work and self-improvement he became an educated and successful tailor. As owner of an exclusive men's shop in Charing Cross he was by day a servant of the wealthy, by night he read, studied and made friends among the intellectuals including James Mill (father of John Stuart Mill), and Jeremy Bentham.

We know that Place was familiar with the theories of Malthus. He felt however that moral restraint would not work as a way of limiting population, and the fact that he was father of 15 children overwhelmingly manifests this viewpoint. Furthermore, he thought that delayed marriage was no solution either, because it would only lead to increased vice. On the contrary, early marriage had the advantage of reducing the rising incidence of venereal disease, and it would contribute to young couples' achievement of better marital relations. Place thought that large families contributed to the child labor problem, and many economists now agree, noting that the passage of legislation restricting child labor had much to do with limiting the number of children in poorer families.

Place and James Mill discussed extensively what should be done to encourage restriction of population. The first written salvo came from Mill, writing for the *Encyclopaedia Britannica Supplement* in 1818. His remarks were a tentative step for the birth control movement: "And yet, if the superstitions of the nursery were discarded, and the principal of utility kept steadily in

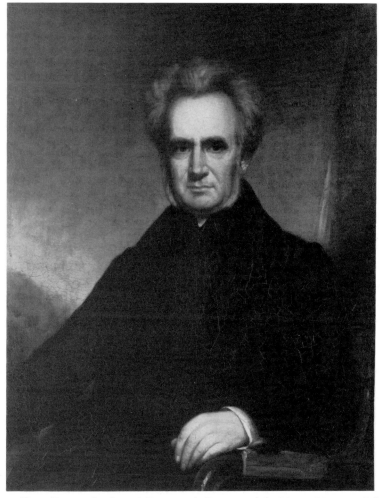

Francis Place. (Painting by Samuel Drummond. Courtesy of the National Portrait Gallery, London)

view, a solution might not be very difficult to be found; and the means of drying up one of the most copious sources of human evil might be seen to be neither doubtful nor difficult to be applied."

Later Mill wrote in encouragement of "prudence" by which he meant that either marriages were to be sparingly contracted, or care taken that children, beyond a certain number, should not be the fruit. (Bentham it was who first suggested contraception for economic reasons, this philosophy being a combination of those of Malthus and Place.)

Place approved of the sentiments expressed by Mill, but as a practical man he felt that explicit instructions were needed rather than general meditations on society. Thus, he wrote and distributed a handbill entitled "To the Married of Both Sexes." In this he advocated withdrawal and/or use of a vaginal sponge. (The sponge was suggested to Place by Jeremy Bentham.) In the later editions of the handbill, Place dropped the suggestion of withdrawal in favor of the sponge option. This caused one reader, identified only as I.C.H., much distress. He felt that "la chamade" (the retreat) was much more genteel, and moreover was not "injurious to the health, nothing offensive to the nicest delicacy."

The condom was in existence at that time but had not been perfected by the use of vulcanized rubber. Wishing to address himself to all segments of society, Place wrote additional handbills: "To the Married of Both Sexes in Genteel Life" and "To the Married of Both Sexes of the Working People." All these handbills had the advantage of being written in the language of the people to whom they were directed. Such suitability of language was not always in evidence in public life. The Lord Chief Justice of England found it necessary to instruct the plaintiff in a rape case: "Woman, you must speak out in plain language that the court and gentlemen of the jury may understand you. You must not mince the matter but call things by their proper names. You must call a spade a spade and not a Thing or a Colly-flower."

The handbills did not stress medical aspects, although Place did mention such terms as "contracted pelvis" and "constitutional disease." It is a matter of record, however, that the author did consult doctors and give some emphasis to the medical viewpoint. One of his good friends was Thomas Walmsley, a medical reformer, the founder of *The Lancet* and for four years its editor. It seems likely that Place was able to give his views some medical background as a consequence of this friendship. Place was generally shunned and castigated on account of these courageous pamphlets. Seeking support from a prominent social worker, Mary Fildes, he received the reaction that the writings were "diabolical filth." He nevertheless continued to work quietly and methodically for a further two decades following publication of the handbills. Perhaps surprisingly, he was never arrested or harassed by the law. Professor Himes says that Place holds a remarkable position in the history of social science, and that "the organizational element which Place introduced was absolutely new so far as present knowledge of the subject is concerned." In his obituary it was said that, "He loved quiet power for the purpose of promoting good ends."

Francis Place spent much time and effort educating his pupils, Richard Carlile, Richard Hassell, and William Campion. Place and his disciples were popularly dubbed Malthusians. Since Malthus never endorsed birth control, it is probably more accurate to class them as Neo-Malthusians. Carlile had on his agenda other items of social reform which he regarded as more important than birth control. Place once commented that Carlile was like the sorcerer's apprentice, off on a mad career of his own, unencumbered by a sense of social restraint concerning sexual matters. This intrepid convert published, in 1826, *Every Woman's Book: What is Love?* The language was crude, and notices in the margins of Place's copy indicate that he found the work unacceptable in its original form. He attempted to persuade Carlile not to publish, however Carlile's commitment to the cause made him forge ahead despite the discomfiture of his mentor. Place was clearly a more profound thinker with a better tactical sense. He was called "the master spring that moves the whole infernal machine."

Every Woman's Book enjoyed a wide circulation. A second edition, abridged by Godfrey Higgins, was subsequently published. Professor Himes says that although the book was coarse and naive it was the first book in the English language that frankly discussed the economic, social and medical aspects of birth control.

While Place was never arrested, Carlile was jailed several times but on the charge of blasphemy rather than obscenity. While in prison, Carlile and his co-workers Hassell and Campion edited and circulated a periodical, "The Newgate Monthly" (from the Newgate prison). Himes dubs them the Newgate Neo-Malthusians, more audacious than astute. An opposing periodical, *The Bull Dog*, was set up. Its sole objective was to castigate Place, Carlile, Bentham and their followers. The accusations and attacks in no way deflected or upset these crusaders; their commitment was resolute and they felt that "truth cannot be slandered."

Several events occurred which had the effect of distracting public attention from the campaign of Place, Carlile and the others. In 1832 a Reform Bill was passed, followed by a new Poor Law in 1834. After the Napoleonic wars, economic problems in England were great but there followed a period of readjustment when such new laws diminished the clamor for social reform and the interest in birth control waned. Professor Himes notes, however, that "there was a quiet penetration of new knowledge throughout all classes of society."

It is perhaps surprising that the French were the first in Europe to practise birth control widely. This was despite the influence of the Roman Catholic Church. Historians have attributed this to the practical way in which French people have traditionally approached financial and sexual matters. Apparently withdrawal was widely practised, and the sponge was also in use.

A contribution to the new movement was made by Dr. H. A. Allbutt, a dignified, well qualified and respected medical practitioner in Edinburgh. He became concerned with the plight of the poor women of that city and in 1887 he published a pamphlet entitled, "The Wife's Handbook." Dr. Allbutt wanted the book to be available to the poor, so he set the price at only sixpence. Critics accused him of catering to the less respectable elements of society. The book dealt principally with prenatal and postnatal care; almost as an afterthought he included a section on contraception. Two important circumstances attended this publication of not particularly novel views. First, the author was a member of the then very conservative Royal College of Physicians of Edinburgh and, secondly, there were included some advertisements for contraceptive materials. As a consequence, Dr. Allbutt's name was removed from the list of Fellows of the Royal College. This raised the good Scottish doctor's ire, so he persisted, and the pamphlet was a huge success, being translated into several languages, and selling hundreds of thousands of copies.

Some believe that the English birth control movement really started when Charles Bradlaugh and Annie Besant printed Dr. Charles Knowlton's *Fruits of Philosophy*. They had organized the Freethought Publishing Company for the sole purpose of reproducing this pamphlet. Wishing to force a court case, they notified the police of the place of distribution. The principals were arrested and the trials took place in 1877–1879. The case was first heard in the Central Criminal Court and then in the High Court before Lord Chief Justice Cockburn. Mrs. Besant delivered an impassioned plea on behalf of the poor people, and the court ruled for the defendants, which gave them the right of publication.

At about the same time, Edward Truelove published a tract, *Moral Physiology*, by J. H. Palmer. This was described by Himes as "chaste and refined, but hortatory." Truelove was a dignified and respectable man of 70, but the Society for the Suppression of Vice nonetheless filed a complaint. Truelove was brought to trial and the first case ended in a mistrial when the jury was unable to agree. The second trial ended in a conviction, and Edward Truelove was sentenced to four months in prison. This caused a storm of protest. The Home Secretary was the recipient of numerous petitions calling for his release, but he refused to act. When Truelove was released on September 12, 1878, there was wild rejoicing.

These two trials, that of Annie Besant and Charles Bradlaugh, and that of Edward Truelove, served to make the distribution of contraceptive material legal in England. This situation contrasted with that prevailing in the United States with its "Comstockery."

Annie Besant next published a pamphlet entitled, "The Law of Population: Its Consequences and Its Bearing Upon Human Conduct and Morals." Her feelings and thoughts were put forcefully:

> "It is useless to preach the limitation of the family, and to conceal the means whereby such limitation may be effected. If the limitation be a duty, it cannot be wrong to afford such information as shall enable people to discharge it. There are various prudent checks which have been suggested, but further investigation of this intricate subject is sorely needed, and it is much to be wished that more medical men would devote themselves to the study of this important branch of physiology."

According to Himes, the little book enjoyed tremendous success, and during the first 12 years of publication 175,000 copies were sold in England alone.

Annie Besant's contribution to the birth control movement comes to an end at this point. Following some sort of divine revelation she became a Theosophist, gave up her Neo-Malthusian views and withdrew the pamphlet. So strong was her new belief that she refused a large sum of money for the copyright.

The Malthusian League formed in 1860 was later disbanded because of public disfavor. Following the Besant/Bradlaugh trial it was re-established and sought to gain support from the heretofore hostile medical profession. The antagonism of the doctors was profound, although it is worth noting that physicians' families were smaller than those of members of other professions. Also decreasing population numbers shown by census figures are evidence that contraception was widely practised, if most surreptitiously. During the period immediately preceding World War I, as well as during the hostilities and immediately afterwards, public opinion was otherwise occupied.

Following the successful outcome of the Besant/Bradlaugh trials, the way was open for action in society to promote birth control measures. Marie Stopes opened a facility in 1921 and went on to make a lifelong commitment to the cause of contraception. Originally a paleobotanist at the University of Manchester, she had met the American campaigner, Margaret Sanger, in 1915 and by 1918 had written a book, *Married Love* and toured the United States as a guest of Mary Ware Dennett and the Voluntary Parenthood

League. Her success in opening a birth control clinic was much aided by the support of her wealthy aircraft manufacturer husband, Humphrey Roe. There was no confrontational opposition to the clinic, and the police made no attempt to close it. Social stigma did, however, become attached to her as symbolized, perhaps, by the Times' refusal to print the announcement of the birth of her son.

By the late 1920s, then, the birth control movement in Britain was well under way. The search was on for good contraceptive methods. A list was drawn up by Professor J. R. Baker of Oxford on behalf of VOLPAR (The Voluntary Parenthood Association), detailing the specifics of the ideal contraceptive method.

1. It should be inexpensive.
2. It should require no special appliance for insertion into the vagina.
3. It should be small.
4. It should be unaffected by the ordinary range of climates.
5. It should neither leave any trace on the skin when handled, nor stain fabrics.
6. It should contain no volatile or odorous substance.

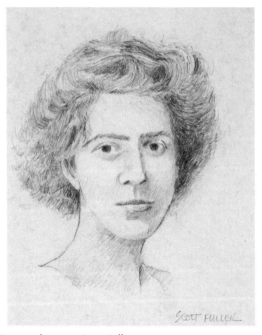

Marie Stopes. (Drawing by artist Scott Fuller)

7. It should be non-irritant to the vagina, cervix or penis.
8. It should be without pharmaceutical effect if absorbed into the bloodstream.
9. It should contain a substance reducing surface tension to ensure the smallest crevices of the folds of the vagina being reached.
10. It should kill sperm at 5/8 or lower concentration in the alkaline and acid test, and the spermicide should diffuse rapidly out of the vehicle into the semen.

Dr. H. M. Carleton, also of Oxford, listed additional goals:

1. To devise methods for evaluating the spermicidal powers of pure substances and/or contraceptive preparations.
2. To investigate the principles underlying the killing of sperm by chemical means.
3. To discover powerful and harmless spermicides.
4. To produce a scientifically satisfactory contraceptive for general use.

THE BIRTH CONTROL MOVEMENT IN THE UNITED STATES

Robert Dale Owen, superintendent of the "free thought" colony established by his father, Robert Owen, in New Harmony, Indiana, was the first to take a substantial public stand on the topic of contraception and population control. How he came to do so was rather by chance. An employee of the colony surreptitiously published an unacknowledged edition of *Every Woman's Book* and Robert Dale Owen was called upon to give his views. Although the text in general was in agreement with his views, Owen felt obliged to go further and set out his own thoughts. In 1831, therefore, he published *Moral Physiology, or a Brief and Plain Treatise on the Population Question*. We should remember that the tradition from the time of the founding of the American colonies was that sexually related matters were regarded as being within the province of the devil. The Puritan mind feared and repressed this subject, with pathological results such as are demonstrated impressively in Nathaniel Hawthorne's *The Scarlet Letter*. As early as Governor Bradford's *History of Plimmoth Plantation* (1630–1650), we find references to "the evils" of contraception, and when we consider the reactionary role of Anthony Comstock in the 19th century, the Puritan inheritance will be unmistakable.

Robert Dale Owen's education had been extensive; he had studied in

Switzerland and travelled throughout Europe. In France, he learned that coitus interruptus was widely practised and that the physicians did not consider it harmful and, as a birth control measure, it was effective. Strangely, he considered the sponge ineffective and the condom expensive and unesthetic. The tract which he published caused him some embarrassment, especially since he was running for a seat in the Indiana Assembly, but despite some opposition he won the support of the local clergy and went on to win the election.

Owen made an important convert in Charles Knowlton (1800–1850). Knowlton was a graduate of Dartmouth (then New Hampshire Medical Institution), and he differed from Owen in that he considered post-coital douching a superior method of contraception. Although Dr. Knowlton maintained a successful medical practice, he was prosecuted three times. The first time he was given a small fine but no sentence; the second time he spent three months in jail; the third trial was nol-prossed. Professor Reed notes that when the English free-thinkers, Annie Besant and Charles Bradlaugh, were prosecuted in England for reprinting "Fruits" in 1877, their well-publicized trial did much to gain support for the birth control movement in the United States.

Early in the development of the movement, a fiery, reactionary figure intervened, one who led a lifelong campaign against all forms of sexual vice as he defined it, and contraceptive practices and ideas were included in his wide-ranging anathema.

Anthony Comstock was born in New Canaan, Connecticut on March 7th, 1844, one of 10 children. His father owned a large farm and was reasonably well off. The greatest influence on Comstock's life was that of his mother, a strict Puritan, and although she died when he was only 10 years old, her influence was with him for the rest of his life. It is quite likely that she contributed unwittingly to his moralistic excesses but, in any event, his character was molded into that of a rigid, bigoted and remorseless crusader. He was not easy on himself, as he harbored many self-doubts and was constantly worried about his own sins. He raided a saloon for the first time when he was 18. According to his biographers, Brown and Leech, he never grew up. They are of the opinion that his religion was "that of Paul, but on occasion and wholly without intent he robs Paul to play Peter Pan."

The war between the States started while Comstock was in high school. After his brother was killed at Gettysburg, he left school to enlist in the Seventeenth Connecticut Volunteers. He saw almost no combat but spent his time on guard duty and proselytizing his fellow soldiers, with whom he

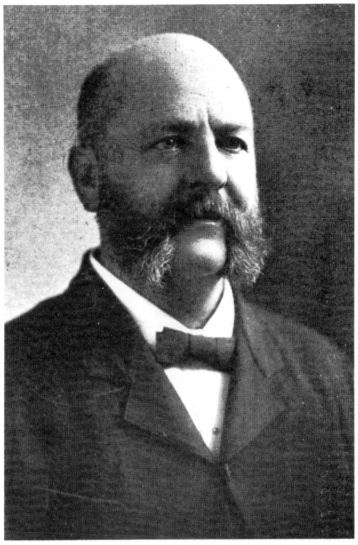

Anthony Comstock. (From *Anthony Comstock: Roundsman of the Lord*, H. Brown and M. Leech, A. & C. Boni, New York, 1927)

was not popular. One illustrative anecdote reveals his dedication to principle. Each soldier was issued a whiskey ration. Comstock dramatically poured his on the ground; he would neither drink it himself nor let another have it. He wrote in his diary that he desired "to govern myself and do all things decently."

After the war he became a dry goods salesman. His personal life was very conservative. His wife was a plain woman 10 years his senior. He wore only black suits complete with black tie, and his only change was to substitute a white tie at Christmas!

After moving to New York, he became aware of the licentiousness of life there and he resolved to do what he could to abolish vice. He obtained the sponsorship of the YMCA and became a one-man vice squad. In time, he obtained the backing of many influential and wealthy men including J. P. Morgan, Kiliaen Van Rensselaer, William Dodge and Samuel Colgate.

His methods of obtaining evidence were devious and often underhanded; this lost him much support. For example, he would write requesting contraceptive material, using an assumed feminine name. On one occasion, he and two associates visited a brothel and watched a "demonstration", following which they arrested the participants. Again, in order to get evidence on the abortionist and purveyor of contraceptives, Madam Restell, Comstock told a sad story of poverty and an unwanted pregnancy. Believing him, she agreed to perform an abortion on his wife, whereupon he had her arrested. She was a dignified lady of 60 years of age and the thought of prison led her to suicide. Much criticism was heaped upon Comstock as a consequence of this episode. His reply was "a bloody ending for a bloody life". He apparently suffered no remorse. Editorials became increasingly critical of his methods. At one meeting, a clergyman asked him three questions, "Did you ever use decoy letters or false signatures? Did you ever sign a woman's name when writing a letter? Did you ever try to make a person sell you forbidden wares and then use the evidence against them?" The answer to all these questions was "Yes".

To Comstock the emerging birth control movement was evil. In no cause did he show a more passionate zeal than in the fight against the purveying of contraceptive remedies or devices. He had been able to obtain legislation banning the use of the US postal service for obscene material. The proscription included contraceptive information or equipment. Some time later the manufacturer of a douche syringe won a court battle, following which he renamed the apparatus the Comstock Bulb. Comstock's biographers assert that he was apparently incapable of believing that any person could be sincerely devoted to the cause of birth control. He considered the purveyors of birth control equipment to be abortionists, and he was also quite unable to distinguish between, on the one hand, medical publications dealing with reproductive processes and, on the other, pornography. He stated that the use of contraceptives made "a brothel of the home". To the horror of his faithful supporter, Samuel Colgate, it was discovered that a pamphlet advertising Vaseline recommended its use as a contraceptive. Needless to say, he quickly ordered deletion of that part of the advertisement.

In 1913, two years before his death, Comstock said in an interview, "In the forty-one years I have been here, I have convicted enough to fill a passenger train of sixty-one coaches, containing sixty passengers each, and the sixty-first almost full". He sounds like a military commander giving an account of the enemy dead. He goes on, "I have destroyed 160 tons of obscene material". As we look back, Comstock appears a fanatical and unattractive figure who, as his biographer says, "set his shoulders granite-like in the way of much truth and much beauty". Some judge that he had a prurient mind, and his intense public activity was fuelled by a personal need to satisfy guilt. He was undoubtedly immoral and inconsistent in his methods of pursuit of vice. Equally certain is the fact that this campaigner, in hindsight both menacing and ridiculous, obscured and delayed the development of the birth control movement in the United States.

Late in his career as a vice vigilante, Anthony Comstock came in conflict with the work of Margaret Higgins Sanger, who is generally credited with being the founder of the birth control movement in the United States. Sixth of 11 children, she seems to have received distinct influences from her parents that helped form her character as "woman rebel". Her father, a professional stonecutter, she describes as a "philosopher, a rebel, and an artist". Irish and agnostic, he settled his family in a largely Roman Catholic area in Corning, New York, and was undaunted by the ensuing ostracizing by his conservative neighbors. His daughter's courageous independence probably developed partly in response to his strongmindedness, or may have been a matter of direct inheritance. The mother, however, was quite different; she was a frail woman who died of tuberculosis at 48. Margaret Sanger felt that the excessive sexual demands and the frequent pregnancies that resulted weakened her mother and contributed to her death. From one parent came the force to carry through as an isolated campaigner; from the other, Margaret Sanger received a deep sense of the sort of female victim on whose behalf she was working.

Margaret Sanger's particular vocation came to her as she followed her work as a nurse. She attended the sick in the tenements of the lower east side of New York, where she was much moved by the plight of the poor, especially the women. The population of the area was made up mostly of European immigrants who knew nothing of birth control, so pregnancies were frequent. In desperation, many of the distraught women resorted to

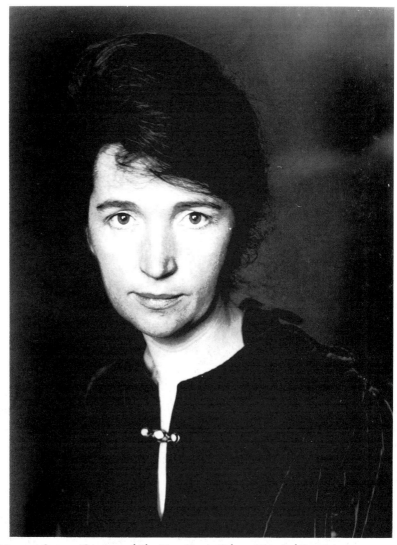

Margaret Sanger. (Courtesy of The New Haven Colony Historical Society)

the dangerous practice of abortion, and the morbidity and mortality was staggering. One such patient, Sadie Sacks, particularly evoked Margaret's sympathy. Following the delivery of yet another child, she implored the physician to tell her how to avoid future pregnancies. His reply was, "Just tell your husband to sleep on the roof". This flippancy enraged Margaret, and her feelings were deepened when, several months later, she attended

Sadie following an abortion which caused a mortal infection. Margaret said the experience of seeing Sadie die changed her life. In her autobiography she described her feelings. She left the squalid quarter and

"walked and walked through the hushed streets. When I finally arrived home and let myself quietly in, all the household was sleeping. I looked out my window and down upon the dimly lighted city. Its pains and griefs crowded in upon me, a moving picture rolled before my eyes with photographic clearness. Women writhing in travail to bring forth little babies; the babies themselves naked and hungry, wrapped in newspapers to keep them from the cold; six-year-old children with pinched, pale, wrinkled faces; old people in concentrated wretchedness, pushed into gray and fetid cellars, crouching on stone floors, their small scrawny hands scuttling through rags, making lamp shades, artificial flowers, white coffins, black coffins, coffins, coffins interminably passing in never-ending succession. The scenes piled up one upon another. I could bear it no longer. As I stood there the darkness faded. The sun came up and threw its reflection over the roof tops. It was the dawn of a new day in my life also. I was resolved to seek out the roots of the evil, to do something to change the destiny of mothers to whom miseries were as vast as the sky."

Following this episode she decided to abandon her general nursing career

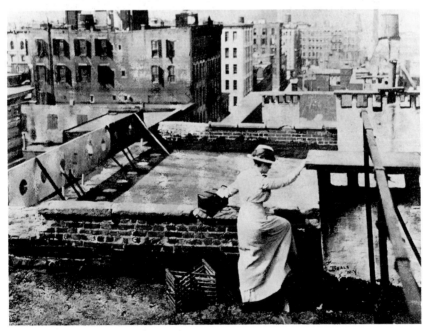

A nurse visiting the poor in the New York tenements, 1908. (Courtesy of the Museum of the City of New York)

and to devote her attention to the birth control cause. While she was in nursing school she had married William Sanger, an architect and painter, and after a brief period in suburbia they returned to New York City and became part of the "bohemian" group. Margaret Sanger vigorously set about her intellectual development in general, and in particular she began to research the literature on contraception. Searches in the Boston Public Library, The Library of Congress and the library of the New York Academy of Medicine produced almost no information on contraception. As her ideas developed. principally in response to her own observation and thinking, she soon came to the conclusion that birth control was far superior to abortion. The sight of women lined up on Saturday nights, sometimes as many as 100, to obtain $5.00 abortions, horrified her, as she was keenly aware of the risk of death.

Ideologically, Margaret Sanger soon adopted socialist orientation. She and her husband became involved in the Ferrer School (named after the Spanish anarchist) which included on its faculty such people as Will Durant, Lincoln Steffens, Clarence Darrow and George Bellows. The New York Times characterized the school as a "hot-bed of radicalism". Strict Marxism, however, did not gain her allegiance. Her friend, Emma Goldman, attending in 1900 a secret meeting in Paris of the Neo-Malthusian Congress, encountered unexpected opposition to birth control from Marxists; the argument was that any reduction in the birth rate of the working class would inevitably diminish that class's political power and prospects. Rather than Marx, Margaret Sanger looked to the Finnish anthropologist, E. A. Westermach, who asserted that from the beginning of recorded history (and probably before) women had sought to limit the number of their children. This was the sort of historical force that Margaret Sanger could wholeheartedly commit herself to.

One of her first contributions to the public debate on contraception was an article entitled, "What Every Girl Should Know." What happened when she tried to mail the pamphlets made clear the type of resistance that existed in United States society — a society that was capable of such a high degree of tolerance of Anthony Comstock. Under the title, "What Every Girl Should Know," a postal official had written "NOTHING."

In 1913 Sanger travelled to Europe to see what she could learn about birth control clinics there. When she returned in early 1914, she brought with her formulae for douche solutions and pessaries. In March, 1914, she published "The Woman Rebel," the masthead slogan of which was "No Gods; No Masters." The subject matter dealt principally with the liberation of women and their right of control over their own bodies. The first issues avoided direct contraceptive information because of the Comstock Law. In the August issue there appeared an article on assassination, the aim of which was to dare the authorities to prosecute. The gauntlet was picked up, the challenge accepted and a date for trial set. In the delay, Margaret Sanger left for Europe, her children and their father remaining behind. Before leaving she had prepared a pamphlet on "Family Limitation," and in her absence an agent of Comstock's vice squad tricked Bill Sanger into giving him a copy. The hope was that when faced with a jail sentence, William Sanger would divulge Margaret's whereabouts. Sanger refused and he consequently spent 30 days in jail. Comstock contracted pneumonia during the trial and died shortly thereafter. While her mother was in Europe, the Sanger's child, Peggy, died of pneumonia. Margaret Sanger harbored a burden of guilt for the remainder of her life, but she refused to allow personal tragedy to stop her work. She demanded a trial on the "Family Limitation" issue and the charges were dropped, even though she refused to promise not to break the law again.

In support of her pamphlets she embarked on speaking tours which made the most of her dramatic flair. She astounded and shocked audiences and seized headlines; at one point she was jailed in Portland, Oregon.

On October 16, 1916, her first birth control clinic in the United States opened in the Brownsville community of Brooklyn. Leaflets advertising the opening were distributed in Yiddish, Italian and English. The clinic was closed down after only 10 days when an undercover policewoman purchased a $2.00 pessary. During the short time of operation, the remarkable number of 488 women were seen. Margaret Sanger and her sister, Ethel Byrne, were arrested in connection with the clinic's allegedly illegal activity and each was sentenced to 30 days in jail. With characteristic toughness, Margaret Sanger resisted being fingerprinted and for a time refused to eat, drink or wash. On release, she marched triumphantly to the prestigious Plaza Hotel, where a luncheon was held in her honor. The entire affair, with appeals and proceedings, lasted until 1918, and it was a further five years before a second birth control clinic was opened.

This time, a physician, Dr Dorothy Bocker, was in charge. Even though Dr Bocker did clinical studies on various methods, Margaret Sanger decided that she did not have sufficient expertise or professional standing to impress the reluctant medical profession. Consequently, Dr Bocker was fired, upon which she avenged herself by taking with her all of the clinical records. Her place was taken for the next three years by Dr Hannah Stone. This doctor

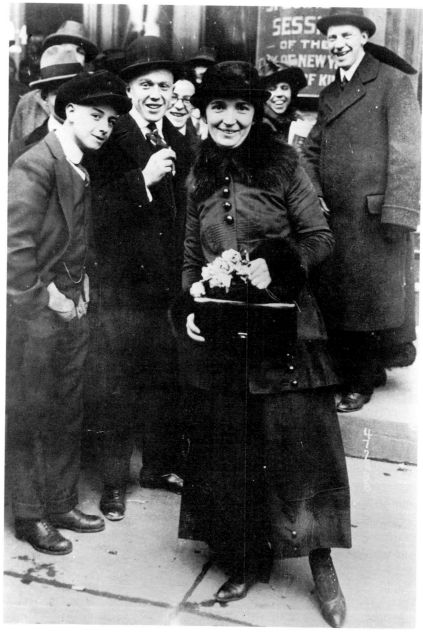

Margaret Sanger on release from jail. (Courtesy of the New Haven Colony Historical Society)

primarily prescribed the diaphragm together with spermicidal jelly. She did a complete survey of the results, covering over 1000 patients, and published her findings in 1928. Even though the preface to the publication was written by Dr Robert Dickinson, a medical practitioner of good standing, the medical profession ignored the venture and its success. When Dr Stone decided to use a type of Japanese pessary and ordered a package of them, the clinic's lawyer, Morris Ernst, was eager to precipitate a test case at law. The clinic was raided, the package seized and he had the opportunity he wanted. The case, *United States vs. One Package*, was tried before Judge Augustus Hand in 1936. Judge Hand noted in his decision that if Congress had possessed knowledge of the dangers of pregnancy and abortion in 1873, the Comstock Law would never have been passed. Further, he observed that the judicial system was in need of education in this matter. His decision opened the mails to contraceptive materials and the back of the Comstock Law was broken at last.

Perhaps, unsurprisingly, such a forthright campaigner as Margaret Sanger made enemies. As early as 1915, while she was in Europe, Mary Ware Dennett formed the National Birth Control League, largely to satisfy a group who wished to distance themselves from the Sangers and their association with supposed anarchists (such as Emma Goldman). Initially, Margaret Sanger sought to work with the new League, but she was told she was not wanted, particularly because her abrasive tactics were not approved of. This conflict was to smoulder on for years.

More fundamental to "the cause" was Margaret Sanger's struggle with the medical establishment. The conflict really developed when she was seeking a physician of stature to work in her first clinic. No reputable gynecologist wanted the job, and a number of factors probably accounted for such reluctance. The medical profession at that time was composed of middle and upper class conservative and moderate physicians — women, ethnic minorities and the common working American were not significantly represented. Margaret Sanger's association with anarchists and liberal organizations made her suspect in the eyes of such conservative practitioners. Furthermore, there was the articulate and persuasive leadership of Dr Morris Fishbein, editor of the influential *Journal of the American Medical Association*. This physician's position concerning birth control was that "no known method is physiologically, psychologically and biologically sound in both principle and practice," and such an attitude carried the allegiance of the majority of American physicians.

Despite such general hostility, Margaret Sanger was able to gain the

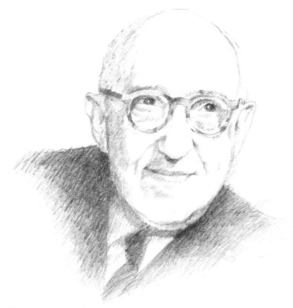

Dr Morris Fishbein. (Drawing by artist Scott Fuller, after an early photograph)

support of a physician of high standing who began the process of enlightenment of the medical profession, a process carried forward later by Dr Robert Latou Dickinson. Margaret Sanger's "find" was a practitioner and academic whose experience had particularly suited him to work in the new clinic. Dr James F. Cooper had left his job as instructor at the Boston University School of Medicine to become a medical missionary in China. He returned to the United States to practise obstetrics in the Boston slums convinced, apparently, that missionary work was needed at home. Dr Cooper answered Dr Fishbein's objections in a book on the technique of contraception.

> "Is it fair, then to ask, have we any 100 percent methods in medicine, or surgery, or serum or vaccine therapy?... The only ethical attitude a physician can take is to guarantee nothing. He can only promise to do his best. This being true, how clearly absurd it is to single out one department of medical practice, namely contraception, for criticism on the grounds that it is not 100 percent perfect, and for that reason regard it with indifference! If all physicians had adopted the same attitude toward every other branch of medicine and surgery, their profession long since would have discontinued its activities. As a matter of fact, there are very few fields indeed in the practice of medicine where such uniformly good results can be obtained as in contraception."

Margaret Sanger saw herself as a woman of destiny (a hobby of hers was to read about great women in history) and there is no doubt that she contributed remarkable thrust to the birth control movement. Historians have placed her within certain ideological movements, but her basic and pragmatic attitude is well expressed by James Reed:

> "William O'Neill has argued that Sanger was the prophet of a new form of domesticity, rendered more palatable by divorce reform and birth control, and finally exposed by Betty Frieden in *The Female Mystique* (1963). Another historian has declared her a prominent figure in the American eugenics movement. She was neither an apologist for marriage nor a eugenicist, but her relationship to both feminism and the eugenics movement was complex. While she shared values with other feminists and eugenicists, she always maintained her distance, insisting that birth control was the essential first step in any rational plan for freeing women or to enable them to breed a better race. She took help wherever she could get it, but the demands of her cause came first, and co-operation did not reach beyond additional justifications for spreading contraceptive practice."

As mentioned earlier, Robert Dickinson played a major role in involving the American medical profession in the birth control movement. Despite being a devout Episcopalian, Dr Dickinson never viewed contraception or sterilization as sinful or a violation of nature. His influence on the national scene began when he was President of the American Gynecologic Society; from this position he made public efforts to support the cause of birth control. His initial address as President was characteristically controversial and committed: "Sexual Counselling and Contraception."

Robert Dickinson was not, however, initially in harmony with the efforts of Margaret Sanger and other birth control campaigners such as Emma Goldman. While he was suspicious of the brash publicity-manipulating behavior of the popular campaigners, he also realized that the medical profession needed to become involved if it was to gain control of some sort over the movement in general. He refused Margaret Sanger's first invitation to participate but reconsidered when he saw that a major opportunity existed for scientific clinical studies. Also, he was aware of the continuing threat posed by Comstock's heir, John Sumner, who might take advantage of false steps in the birth control campaign to whip up public distrust and develop legal problems.

The second time Margaret Sanger approached Robert Dickinson, he didn't hesitate to accept, and he played an important role on a maternal research council funded by the Rockefellers. Operating within the birth control movement, Robert Dickinson significantly drew the medical establishment

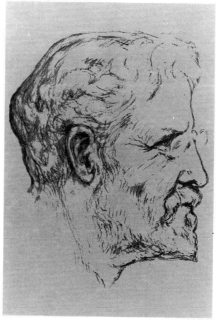

Robert Latou Dickinson. Self portrait (Courtesy of Ortho Pharmaceutical Corporation)

into that controversial field and facilitated its progressive legitimation. His calm and reasonable approach to the social and medical aspects was responsible for the slow penetration of scientific objectivity in most circles. "In all marriages whatever, except in marriages where both partners are ascetic, sterile or impotent, birth control and the mechanism of love loom large as techniques of happiness. Honoring all honorable acts of love means teaching them. There in nature is no better guide than other works of art. No act of life is without a technique training."

Robert Dickinson and Margaret Sanger in their continuing association did not always see eye to eye. He disliked her flamboyant ways, but they were nevertheless able to work together. When she was severely criticized by the new American Birth Control League, Dr Dickinson came swiftly to his colleague's defense. "Mrs. Sanger is the symbol, the international figure, possessed of ability to beget enthusiasm for this work beyond anyone else whatever. She has a way of delivering goods which makes our other groups appear somewhat as though mechanisms of organization, conformities, and fear of the medical guild were their main concerns."

When he died in 1950, Robert Dickinson had not lived to see the end

CONTRACEPTION: A MEDICAL REVIEW OF THE SITUATION*

FIRST REPORT OF THE COMMITTEE ON MATERNAL HEALTH OF NEW YORK

BY ROBERT L. DICKINSON, M.D., F.A.C.S., NEW YORK CITY

THE medical profession has scant knowledge on which to base advice on control of conception. The gist of what is known is here given, together with an account of the attempts to secure clinical data.

As the objects of the committee were stated in this Journal last March (vol. vii, p. 339), it need only be said here that its scientific investigation of contraception—a section of its study of sterility and fertility—is under the complete medical control of a considerable group of representative physicians; that sponsoring the study was voted for in a questionnaire by the New York Obstetrical Society, and that an endorsement was given by the Public Health Committee of the Academy of Medicine.† This work is deemed to be a complete review of the medical literature; personal inspections of birth control clinics and their records; critical collection of foreign experience and American practice; an agreement on general medical indications; consideration of technic; standards for acceptable case histories and the collection and analysis of these; chemical and animal experimentation, and the setting of (and remuneration for) necessary research problems, laboratory and clinical, bearing on fertility and sterility,—all clinical work, when undertaken here, to be within the interpretation of our law[30] that sanctions contraception only "to cure or prevent disease."

Deeming its most important duty to be the organization of a series of impartial, well-studied clinical tests, and believing that these should be made in responsible institutions, the committee made appropriations of $300 each to six out-patient departments in order to add to its collection of adequate case records. It is also searching for hospital cases since an inspection was made of the cards in one doctor's office covering more than a thousand patients for whom she had placed the "wishbone stem," and the finding, in several institutions, histories of serious damage done by this implement. Moreover the committee is trying to overcome the difficulty involved in securing and providing the supplies required in order to study certain claims.

Need of Investigation by the Medical Profession.—The data concerning contraception which can be brought together at this time are only

---

*Read at the Forty-ninth Annual Meeting of the American Gynecological Society, May 15, 1924.

†The American Gynecological Society, at the meeting at which this paper was presented, voted to appoint a committee to cooperate.

First page of a landmark article by Dr Robert Latou Dickinson. The first American physician of stature to endorse contraception. (Courtesy of Ortho Pharmaceutical Corporation)

February 20, 1942

Mr. Robert L. Dickinson
360 East 50th Street
New York City

Dear Robert L:

It was most kind of you to write me as to your
feeling in accepting "Planned Parenthood". I would not
object to the term "Planned Parenthood" if it were a more
aggressive and challenging title, but it irks my very soul
and all that is Irish in me to acquiesce to the appeasement
group that is so prevalent in our beloved organization. We
will get no further because of the title; I assure you of
that. Our progress up to date has been because the Birth
Control movement was built on a strong foundation of
truth, justice, right, and good common sense.

The contribution, dear Robert L, that you and I
have made has been adhering to the policy of placing
instruction for all in the hands of the medical profession.
In spite of Mrs. Dennett's ability and her popular appeal
to the free-speechers, in spite of her opposition to medical instruction for the masses, our stand was the right
stand, and consequently has won. What we must do now is
to strike while the iron is hot. By this I mean that the
present administration in Washington is friendly, not only
to us but is definitely out to give the "under-dog" knowledge and opportunity to better himself, and Birth Control
does just that.

If you, dear Robert, can now concentrate all
your efforts, supported by the prestige of your national
reputation, upon the A.M.A. and county and state medical
groups, bringing the A.M.A. up to date with the public
health crowd, you will indeed have won for the movement
its final victory.

It's nice that you live near 501. I sincerely
hope that you are in your usual excellent health. And
thank you so much for your good letter.

Cordially, ever

Letter from Margaret Sanger to Robert L. Dickinson. (Courtesy of Ortho Pharmaceutical
Corporation)

altogether of the "hush and pretend." He had, however, been the person most responsible for the acceptance of birth control by the medical establishment. This was essential, for without it clinical studies and research in reproductive physiology and pharmacology would have been conducted under a cloud of professional antipathy.

The birth control movement made progress in the United States as a result of a stiff struggle over 100 years and more. If Anthony Comstock typifies melodramatic and fiery resistance to contraception, the treatment of the issue in the state of Connecticut can be taken to represent the many instances of the slow legal struggle that took place throughout the nation.

Connecticut was the last state to legalize the operation of Planned Parenthood clinics. There were several reasons for this slowness to fall in with the movement of the times. Native son Anthony Comstock's anti-vice campaigns had a lingering influence. In addition to the "Comstock effect", the state legislature was controlled by urban politicians who were largely Roman Catholic, and that church had set its face against birth control in any form. Traditional New England Puritans were similarly resistant. Comstock's federal law banning the use of the postal service for the sending of "obscene" material was passed by Congress in 1873; a corresponding bill went through the Connecticut legislature in 1879. This latter bill was more wide-reaching in that it forbade the use of any drug or device to prevent conception. In 1923 the 1879 bill received its first challenge: an amendment to the birth control law was introduced in the legislature. A meeting took place in Hartford for those supporting the move and Margaret Sanger addressed the assembled supporters. Shortly thereafter, Mrs Thomas Hepburn (mother of the famous actress) and her friends formed the Connecticut Birth Control Clinic, the first one in the United States. Mrs Hepburn, wife of a prominent physician, said, "I believe that all women want children. It is a maternal instinct. But they also want to take care of their children properly and educate them. It is agony of the first order when they can't do these necessary things." The 1879 legislation, however, was not overturned.

From 1935 to 1939 Birth Control Clinics were opened in several locations in the state. Supporters felt that their legality would never be challenged and some 9,000 women received help. In 1939, however, state police raided the Waterford Clinic. Two physicians and a nurse were arrested and this action forced the other clinics to close. In 1940, a group of physicians brought suit in the state courts where they were ruled against. Later the case was dismissed by the Supreme Court. Throughout the 1940s and into the 1950s the determined women and their physician supporters continued

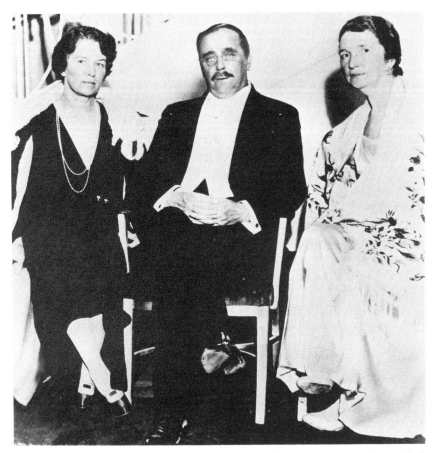

Mrs Thomas Hepburn, H. G. Wells and Margaret Sanger attending a dinner at the Waldorf Astoria Hotel, New York, 1931. (Courtesy of the New Haven Colony Historical Society)

the fight. Yearly efforts to obtain relief through the state legislature were unsuccessful. There was very little opposition in the house of representatives but the senate remained resistant. The majority of senators were unwilling to antagonize the Roman Catholic Church.

In 1961 Estelle Griswald and Professor Lee Buxton (a distinguished professor and Chairman of the Department of Obstetrics and Gynecology at Yale University Medical School) opened a clinic in New Haven, fully expecting to be arrested as a consequence. Both had deep convictions regarding birth control and the wider topic of sex education. Shortly after the clinic opened, a man presented himself and accused Mrs Griswald and

Dr Buxton of "doing the devil's work and getting rich at it". Arrests followed and the case went on to the United States Supreme Court. Yale law professor Thomas Emerson pled the case on March 29 and 30, 1965, and after an agonizing delay the verdict came that the Connecticut birth control law was "unconstitutional". The domination of Comstockian attitudes was at an end.

It is interesting to note, and generally indicative of the climate of opinion in the United States as far as contraception is concerned, that one of the major problems in establishing clinics was the name to be used. Acceptance could not come if the phrase, "birth control", was used; something without *odium sexicum* was needed. The solution was the name, "Family Planning Clinic", and it achieved acceptance successfully. The name implies that each couple may have as many children as they wish, and therefore conveys no prejudice against fertility and large families. In addition, the name does not necessarily imply contraception. This verbal sleight of hand achieved what was intended in soothing minds sensitive to the irreligious and unnatural potential aspects of contraception. Perhaps we shouldn't be surprised to learn that Margaret Sanger, in her fearless directness, was against the new and pragmatic name!

BIRTH CONTROL AND THE EMANCIPATION OF WOMEN

The birth control movements in Britain and the United States inevitably contributed to the wider movement of female emancipation. Detailed

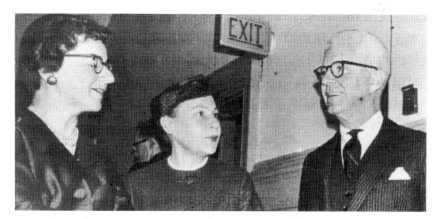

From left to right attorney Catherine Rorabach, Mrs Griswald and Dr Lee Buxton during the Connecticut trial

commentary on this major relationship is not possible here, but some general pointers should be offered in order to suggest just how fundamental the birth control struggle was to the progressive emancipation of women over the last 100 years.

From early times women were held back from full participation in the economic, intellectual and political life of Western societies. It would be a distortion to suggest that the insistent physiological features of menstruation and pregnancy were alone responsible for the restricted contribution made by women to many of the major processes of society. Religious, gender-genetical, other physiological, and economic factors, among others, were all most likely involved to some extent in the holding back of women from exercising their right to be human beings first and women second. Whatever the combination of forces which restricted women for centuries, the success of birth control campaigners contributed strongly to the growing capacity of women to realize their potential within modern society.

The birth control movement, through its raising to the public notice of the facts of human reproduction, helped women struggle clear from a difficult and contradictory role within sexual mythology. Victorian middle-class women were expected to be asexual in behavior, while many of their lower-class sisters were to be easy and sluttish. Respectable Victorian men were acknowledged to have need of both. Women thus were burdened, through male fantasy and power, with an insupportable hybrid role — both Eve and the Blessed Virgin Mary. Birth control campaigning drew attention to the amoral, scientific facts of human reproductive behavior and enabled women to begin to escape from circumstances engineered by wish-fulfillment and fear.

Perhaps progress in birth control methods and acceptability brought most obvious freedom and relief from the physical point of view. Traditionally, women had been under continuous physical threat on account of uncontrolled childbearing — Margaret Sanger's patient, Sadie Sacks, is an example. Caught between the church-sanctified libido of the husband and the morbid fear of the pain and danger of repeated pregnancies, it is not surprising that women usually had little energy to participate more widely in society. Control of the number of pregnancies, greater understanding of the process of childbearing, the coming forward of methods and attitudes which alleviated the pain aspect — together such factors reduced the physical burden placed on the sex that carries the child until it is independently viable. Additionally, modern-day science is enabling further control through the introduction of hormone treatment to ease the menopause and control some of its otherwise abrupt and serious consequences.

The loss of what was often a fearful mental preoccupation with the reproductive function has certainly provided psychological benefits for women. Birth control has offered some freedom which has encouraged the exercise of choice and all the self-development associated with such choice. The traditional self-protective habits of subservience or deceitful subversion are on the wane, and women's personal control over their bodies is largely responsible for this improved mental orientation.

Socially, there has been gain too, as everyone is aware. Released from permanent child-centered household existence, women have become free to explore new roles in society; they have tested long latent abilities; they have shaken some male monopolies and led men to widen the scope of their life options too. Advances in birth control again must be seen as having cleared the space for the new freedom.

The most dramatic manifestation of female emancipation in the 20th century was probably the Suffragette Movement, but it is arguable that the availability of safe and effective contraceptives has done more of substance for the emancipation of women than did the achievement of suffrage.

7

Methods of Contraception before the Pill

Of course, the Birth Control Movement in Britain and the United States was dependent in many ways on the development and acceptability of suitable contraceptive methods. This chapter sets out to review the various methods and devices for contraception which were current before the revolutionary introduction of hormonal methods.

ABORTION

This is one of the oldest remedies for unwanted pregnancy, and it is still used under a number of circumstances. In pre-literate and ancient times one of the chief methods of population control was that of abortion and infanticide. This method was resorted to when war, famine, disease and desertion of the aged were insufficient. There were some civilizations that did not support abortion however; the tenth-century Persian, Rhazes, listed 24 methods of contraception, but none involved abortion, suggesting that this civilization found abortion an unacceptable remedy. Aristotle, on the other hand, approved of abortion and death by exposure of defective infants. Other ancient Greeks recommended abortion under circumstances such as contracted pelvis, poor maternal health and pregnancy caused by rape or adultery. Given the procedures used and the inability at the time to control infection, the decision to abort on grounds of health must have been an awkward one. Whether plant substances or surgical techniques were used, infection and ineffectiveness must have been common. Whether the anciently approved root of the mallow was used, or the more modern "slippery elm", the risk of infection and ensuing death would have been high.

    The incidence of abortion declined during the Middle Ages, especially in Europe. This was largely because of the anathema of the Roman Catholic church. The practice was not, however, wholly eliminated. Professor Himes comments on the existence of folk abortifacients of the period details of which were furtively passed from one person to another, so that an accurate listing of what was then practised is now not possible. Records do exist, however, indicating that marjoram, myrtle, root of worm fern and others were in use. All such would have been relatively ineffective.

Until quite recently, abortions have been performed secretly and usually illegally. In Europe, the Eastern Block of nations was the first to legalize abortion. Only three years after the 1917 Revolution the Soviet Union made abortion legal, and the other communist countries followed later. The practice also became a major population-controlling method in the Orient. By 1950, for example, there were 170,000 abortions being performed in Japan annually.

The story in Britain has been different. There were certainly many illegal abortions done in that country, although in 1955 there were only 66 cases prosecuted. This figure represented only the tip of the iceberg. By 1968, however, the laws had been liberalized.

The United States moved later but implementation was swifter. The last word has not yet been said, as the "Right to Life" movement and the present Administration are for repeal of the Abortion Act. A majority, though certainly not all physicians, agree with former Vice-president Nelson Rockefeller who said "Repeal would not end abortions, it would only end abortions under safe and supervised medical conditions".

The uncontrolled situation in the Central and South American countries is staggering; although accurate figures are not available, estimates of illegal abortions run into the millions.

It is a conservative estimate that every year nearly one and a half million women in the United States and 40 million world-wide have abortions. Lack of access to effective birth control measures must be responsible for a high proportion of these abortions.

The subject of abortion remains an emotionally and philosophically charged issue. What should be done about a young girl pregnant as a result of rape or incest? Countless instances arise where conflicting rights require to be mediated and extremes of human feeling are involved. Even when an abnormal child seems very possible and abortion appears a justifiable escape from suffering, even under such circumstances certainty is elusive, as the apocryphal Beethoven example suggests. One doctor to another: "About the termination of a pregnancy, I wish your opinion. This was the mother's fifth pregnancy. The father was syphilitic, the mother tuberculous; of four children born the first was blind, the second died, the third was deaf and dumb, the fourth tuberculous. What would you have done?" Second doctor answers: "I would have terminated the pregnancy". First doctor: "Then you would have murdered Beethoven".

Despite the terrible problems associated with it, abortion remains a major method in use for population control. It is not a preferred method, certainly, but it will not easily go away. Contemporary anti-abortion trends in some Western countries do not seem to represent progress. In the United States if the "Right to Life" movement persuades the Supreme Court to reverse its previous decision, the back-alley will once again become the surgical suite, with all its dangers to the mother's health and the new life itself.

The answer, in ideal terms, is avoidance of the need for abortion. The majority of teenage girls having sex for the first time are not protected against becoming pregnant so early in their lives, and better sex education would cut down the number of unwanted pregnancies. Moral and prudent behavior cannot be legislated for, but well calculated sex education can lead young people to act more self-consciously in the interest of their own happiness and that of possible new human beings.

PROLONGED LACTATION

Since ancient times it has been recognized that women tended to be relatively infertile during the postpartum period. This was noted especially if lactation was prolonged. It was not until recently, however, that statistical methods were used to study this phenomenon. Dr Alan Guttmacher reported on this in 1958, estimating that the average duration of amenorrhea in the absence of lactation was about two months. This was followed by another two months of two anovulatory cycles for a total of four months. If, on the other hand, the infant was breast fed, then the period of relative infertility could extend for as long as nine months.

Lactation does not, however, invariably prevent ovulation, as the late Robert Greenblatt has pointed out. Furthermore, there is a widespread practice of sexual abstention during lactation which may contribute to the low conception rate at that time. That the lactating woman could become pregnant was recognized by Rabbi Eleazor in the first century AD. He condoned withdrawal by the husband during intercourse in the lactating period, commenting tactfully that the husband could "thresh inside and winnow outside".

On a world-wide scale, prolonged lactation is probably the method of birth control most in effect. In poorer countries, where bottle-feeding is not a practicality, prolonged lactation is inevitable and temporary birth control operates as a consequence. Of course, the limits of this method are obvious; lactation can only continue for a relatively short period in comparison with a woman's total period of potential fertility.

COITUS INTERRUPTUS

There is no doubt that coitus interruptus has been widely practised ever since it was recognised that semen was essential for fertilization. The Bible provides a famous early recorded example, even if the episode has frequently been misinterpreted as a condemnation of masturbation. The story can be summarized as follows.

"Onan's brother, Er, died so Judah said unto Onan: 'Go in unto thy brothers' wife and perform the duty of a husband unto her, and raise up seed to thy brother', and Onan knew that the seed would not be his; and it came to pass, whenever he went in unto his brother's wife, that he used to spill it on the ground lest he should give seed to his brother, and the thing which he did was evil in the sight of the Lord; and he slew him also".

Commentators have not noticed that the sin implied is failure to follow the marriage law that requires a man to have children by his deceased brother's wife, raising them in his brother's name. Onan's reason for not wishing to do so is not clear, and this potential for ambiguity has made possible the wrong interpretation.

It is worth noting that coitus interruptus has been condemned by the Roman Catholic Church as firmly as any of the more interventionary means of preventing conception. This topic was thoroughly covered by Saint Thomas Aquinas in *Suma Theologica*. Whether or not coitus interruptus is a sin, it is far from an ideal method of contraception, as the late Robert Greenblatt has commented. He says, "Coitus interruptus, a primative and elementary form of contraception, still is practised widely. It is a practice that weighs on the conscience of man, and does violence to an act that should engender tenderness, fulfilment and the sublimest of emotional nuances. A great deal of illness among women, manifested in a dozen ways, may be traced to such and other unsatisfactory sexual experiences".

Similar to coitus interruptus is coitus reservatus. The Chinese, in ancient times, practised this method of contraception. When pregnancy was not desired, the sexual act was performed with intromission and coital movements until the point when emission seemed imminent. Then movements were stopped and detumescence occurred intravaginally. It is difficult to believe that this method was very reliable, and Robert Greenblatt's reservations concerning the psychological effects of coitus interruptus must apply as strongly in the case of coitus reservatus.

John Humphrey Noyes' commune near Oneida in New York practised coitus reservatus. The commune was based on a religious doctrine which they called "perfectionism". Noyes believed in the Galton doctrine of eugenics, and in implementation of this belief, he established a breeding committee which had the authority to arrange matings. They named this system "stirpiculture". Selection was based more on religious piety than on intelligence, health, strength or background. In 1848, Noyes made this statement:

> "We are not opposed to procreation, but we are opposed to involuntary procreation. We are opposed to excessive and, of course, oppressive procreation, which is almost universal. We are opposed to random procreation, which is unavoidable in the marriage system. But we are in favor of intelligent, well-ordered procreation — we believe the time will come when involuntary and random procreation will cease, and when scientific combination will be applied to human generation as freely and successfully as it is to that of other animals".

Noyes rejected other methods of contraception such as the condom, the sponge and the douche. Regardless of how bizarre Noyes' ideas may seem to us now, studies indicate that infant mortality was low, and the health and longevity of the community members was better than average. In 1921, Edwin Kopf, statistician for the Metropolitan Life Insurance Company, studied the stirpicultural group. The mortality rates were only 32% of a typical rural community and 24% of the total New York State experience.

Public opinion forced abandonment of the community, but not before some valuable lessons had been learned. The verdict of Robert Dickinson (see Chapter Six) was rendered in a letter to Dr Hilda H. Noyes: "The Oneida Community experience is, as far as I can judge, the only long-continued group of intelligent people using a single method, combined with physical examinations to check up the effects on health — Further, I am informed by a reliable source that four-fifths of the children were planned". This open-minded and discriminating commentary contrasts with much of the fearful and vituperative opinion that led to the ending of the communal experiment.

Dr Alice B. Stockham, a popular medical writer of the 1880s and 90s and a disciple of Noyes, promoted the practice of coitus reservatus, which she called Karezzo. She asserted that this was the most desirable form of birth control, even though in her book *Karezzo, Parenthood and Tokology*, she mentions other methods, i.e. douche and withdrawal. She labelled as ridiculous the notion that female passiveness would prevent conception. This was a blow on behalf of female emancipation as much as a reputable medical judgement.

Finally, there is what has been termed coitus Saxonicus. This was described in the 14th century by Kappoma in *The Secret of Sexual Disease*. In this technique the woman compresses the man's urethra, blocking the emission of semen which is thereby discharged into the bladder. (In China the same procedure was carried out by the man which seems sensible since he is a better judge of the time of orgasm.)

THE CONDOM

As with many early contraceptive practices the origin of the penile sheath is lost in the mists of ancient history. A tablet from the Egyptian XII dynasty (1350–1200 BC) depicts a protective sheath covering the glans penis. The purpose of this sheath is not certain; it might be an ornament or a talisman (the figure is wearing nothing else), or it might serve to protect the part from trauma, insect bites or tropical diseases such as bilharzia. It could even be a badge of rank or a status symbol.

Some African women employed a hollowed-out okra pod as a vaginal pouch — the female condom. It would appear that this was certainly a contraceptive device. Goat's bladder was used by Roman women in the same way.

That the condom was known in Ancient Rome is revealed in the legend of Minos and Pasiphae, as cited by Himes from an account by Antoninus Liberalis. Prokris, daughter of Erechtheus, left her husband Cephalus because of a dispute. She sought refuge with Minos, the King of Crete. The semen of Milos was said to contain serpents and scorpions. His wife Pasiphae was the daughter of the Sun god and as such was immune to mortal injury. She had not, however, been able to conceive because of the abnormal semen. Prokris slipped a goat's bladder in the vagina, and into this Minos discharged his serpent-bearing semen. Thus rid of the curse, he was able to cohabit with Pasiphae and they eventually were able to have four sons and four daughters.

It seems relatively clear that condoms were in use by men at the time of the Renaissance. Slaughterhouse workers devised condoms made of sausage skins, and Gabrello Fallopia described a linen sheath in a treatise written in 1564. The sheath was in general use in Europe by 1671. In that year Madam de Sevigné, in a letter to her daughter, the Countess of Grinon, knowingly described the condom as "an armor against enjoyment and a spider web against danger".

Casanova de Seingalt (1725–1798) used the condom both as a contraceptive and as a disease preventative. He was, however, reluctant to use the sheath because, as he put it, he did not "like to close himself in" with dead skin! Lest we give him credit for scientific insight in this matter, Casanova also placed faith in three gold balls to be inserted into the vagina. He purchased them from a Genovese goldsmith for approximately one hundred dollars. They would not seem well suited to block the semen as they could easily be dislodged, neither would one expect any spermacidal effect since gold is a very inert metal. Nevertheless, Casanova held that they had served him well for 15 years.

Condoms were apparently in general use in the latter years of the eighteenth century. One finds the following entry in James Boswell's *London Diary* of November 25th, 1762: "I was really unhappy for want of woman. I picked up a girl in the Strand, went into a court with intention to enjoy her in armour, but she had none". In another entry he did use "armour" but both he and the girl found that it diminished the pleasure. On yet another occasion when he felt that he was safe and did not use protection he contracted gonorrhea. Bachaunont's diary, written in 1773, contains the following couplet addressed to a certain ballet dancer. "You know the use of the condom. The condom, my daughter, is the law and the prophet".

The origin of the word "condom" is in doubt. It appeared in a dictionary of London Street Language in 1785 ("condum"). It has been most commonly held that the name came from a Dr Conton, who practised during the reign of Charles II, (1630–1685). The rumor was that as the King became distressed at the number of illegitimate children that he was siring he sought the help of Dr Conton. Others have maintained that the word came from the Latin "condere" and Richter believes that the word is of Persian origin — "rendii" or "kondii", which denotes a vessel made of animal intestine used to store grain. Other names were "armour", "gant des dames", "collette d'assurance", "peau devine" and "chemisette". A writer to Frances Place noted that the woman sometimes insisted on "moucher la chandell" (snuffing the candle — a reference to the use of a condom).

It is doubtful that a Dr Conton ever existed. Suspicion is based partly on the fact that neither Evelyn or Pepys mention such a person in their diaries. However, Finch and Green point out that not all contemporaries were mentioned by those authors, and they cite the French writer P.J. Cabanes who postulated that Dr Conton was so embarrassed to have the sheath named for him that he changed his name.

There is evidence of vigorous and open sale of condoms in the eighteenth century. In 1776, a Mrs Philips of Half Moon Street, London, distributed handbills offering for sale condoms of high quality at her establishment, the Green Cannister. Sometime later, she sold her business to a Mrs Perkins. When she later wished to re-establish her enterprise, a bitter and long-standing feud developed between the two women.

Both national antagonism and moral guilt of some sort are suggested by the way in which the French and the English have informally named the condom after each other. The English have called it "the French letter" while the French refer to "la capote anglaise".

In modern times the condom has become more reliable and acceptable. Goodyear's invention in 1843 of the process of vulcanization of rubber, taken up by Hancock in England a year later, led to the condom becoming more reliably contraceptive and less damaging to sexual satisfaction. Costs of production were also reduced, and later development of latex materials and automation in manufacture improved the product and the ease of its availability. There has been a contemporary upsurge in interest in the condom because of the terrible threat, world-wide, of AIDS. Increased use of the condom would certainly stem the tide of this modern-day plague. The condom, long a contraceptive option, is claiming renewed favor.

THE CAP AND THE DIAPHRAGM

In a treatise written in 1838, Fredrick Adolph Wilde described a rubber cap designed to fit over the cervix. He felt that he had discovered a method more reliable than the condom, the sponge or withdrawal. He perceived that since the size of the cervix differs, the cap should be moulded to the individual. A few years later Mesinga designed a so-called diaphragm that fitted under the pubic bone and covered the cervix. This was soon to replace the cap in popularity and it has proved effective and continues to be used widely.

Perhaps the first recorded use of a diaphragm is found in the memoires

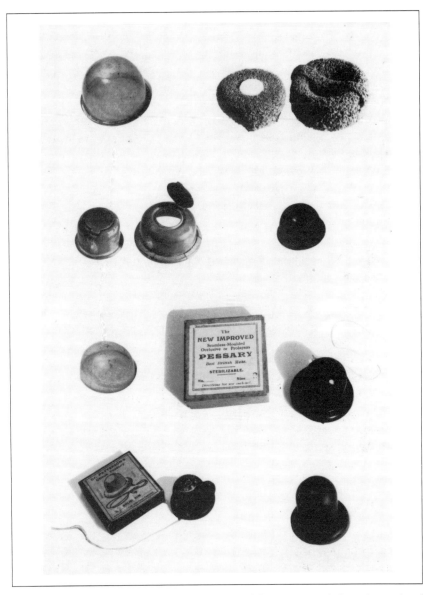

Examples of early contraception devices. (Courtesy of the International Planned Parenthood Federation)

of Casanova. His prescription called for the use of half a lemon, inserted in the vagina and covering the cervix. This method was very likely highly successful because it combined a barrier with a highly spermacidal acid. It was probably as effective as the modern diaphragm used with a spermacidal cream or jelly. The only obstacle was that some instruction was necessary then, as now, in the technique of placement. Also, the correct size was needed. No doubt Cassanova overcame both of these disadvantages because he fashioned the diaphragms himself, and very likely fitted them also.

THE INTRAUTERINE DEVICE

There are records that in ancient times there was undeveloped awareness of this method of contraception. Camel drivers noticed that the usually docile camel became fractious and difficult when pregnant, and it became the practice to prevent pregnancy by inserting small pebbles into the uterus of this important beast of burden. It remains a wonder as to how the originator of this practice learned of its efficacy; also, one wonders why the discovery was not applied in some way to humans.

The first recorded use of the intrautrine device in modern times occurs in the 1920s when Ernst Grafenberg began to experiment. He fashioned handmade, star-shaped devices out of silkworm gut, and in 1928 reported

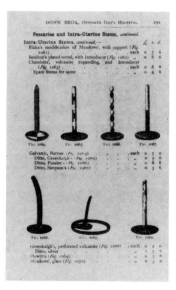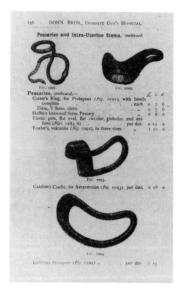

Catalog entries for early pessaries and intrauterine stems. (Courtesy of the International Planned Parenthood Federation)

on his experience with their use as a contraceptive. One complication he observed was frequent expulsion. In order to overcome this he began to use a ring made of silver wire (the so called Grafenberg Ring). Dr Grafenberg went some way in recognizing the problems associated with the insertion and removal of IUDs. His favored technique was to grasp the cervix with a tenaculum following which the cervix was dilated. He also made a thin hook to be used in removal.

The medical profession reacted to Dr Grafenberg's device in characteristic manner; there were those who considered it miraculous and those who condemned it out of hand. Many individual doctors and scientists followed Grafenberg in trying to discover the ideal IUD which would achieve fully reliable contraception and offer no problems associated with placement, retention or removal.

Some practitioners took up the new device enthusiastically only to have doubts later. Dr Norman Haire of London used IUDs for a number of years but apparently became disenchanted because he did not recommend them in his later years. Another early advocate was the Danish physician, Dr J.H. Leunbach. He too condemned the IUD after years of use because of contraception failure and the occurence of intrauterine infections.

Dr Oppenheimer of Israel used both the silkworm gut and silver ring devices extensively. He recorded failure rate of 2.5% per 100 years of exposure and as a result considered the IUD method safe and effective. The Japanese physician, T. Ota, began studying modifications in 1934. He used a ring made of metal or plastic with a flat disc in the center. A colleague, Dr Atsumi Ishihama, reported favorably on a large cohort of patients, noticing no serious complications. In 1962, Drs Herbert Hall and Martin Stone reported on the use of a coil spring made of stainless steel (The Hall Stone Ring). Dr Jack Lippes of Buffalo fashioned a loop made of polyethelene. Dr Birnberg's IUD was a plastic bow.

Following these pioneering feats the Copper T and the Copper 7 IUDs were manufactured on a large scale. One disadvantage remaining was that replacement was required every three years.

Widespread use of IUDs went reasonably well until the A.H. Robbins Company manufactured and distributed the "Dalkon Shield". The composition of the string was such that bacteria had access to the uterine cavity causing infection, often serious and with some fatalities. A not uncommon infection was due to actinomycosis. Many lawsuits were brought against the A.H. Robbins Company and they were forced into bankruptcy. The good standing of the IUD was thrown into doubt and at the present time all IUDs are off the market in the US except one, the progestersert, which contains progesterone, thereby giving added protection. Recently a new copper devise has been reintroduced.

Dr Sheldon Segal points out that the IUD is probably more suited to the developing countries where "logistically complex" oral contraception is less viable. Generally it can be said that the IUD is relatively safe, although some method failures do occur and fall out and infection are real if infrequent problems.

THE SAFE PERIOD

A number of the ancients recognised that there was a fertile time and a non-fertile time in a woman's cycle, even though the process of the ovarian cycle was unknown at the time. Hippocrates, in *De Mortis Mulierium*, said that just before menstruation there was a "safe period". Soranus, on the other hand, thought that the mid cycle was the safe time and the fertile period occurred just before and just after that safe time. Avicenna mentioned a safe period but did not specify the time.

Scientific confirmation of the safe period was a long time in coming. The breakthrough came in 1930 when Ogino in Japan and Knaus in Austria independently determined that ovulation occurred in mid cycle. It became known that basal body temperature rose when ovulation was imminent and, consequently, couples desiring a pregnancy and those wishing not to achieve one have been greatly aided. As a contraceptive method there are weaknesses: the rise in temperature is slight and can vary in time a little; the life span of the male sperm is variable also and this contributes on occasion. Soon after recognition of the temperature rise indicator, physiologists observed a mid cycle change in the character of the cervical mucus. At ovulation time, the thick tenacious mucous plug changes into a clear, thin, watery discharge. Clift in 1936 suggested that this mucus could facilitate sperm penetration.

The Christian church, particularly in the case of Roman Catholicism, has favoured the so called "rhythm method" of contraception where exposure during the mid cycle period is avoided. This method is the only birth control measure endorsed by the Roman Catholic church even now. An early Christian sect, the Abelines (after Abel, the second son of Adam and Eve), had as a major tenet that they remain childless. Normal intercourse was practised, therefore, only during menstruation. This sect must have possessed an early appreciation of the "safe period". The Hebrews apparently understood the time of the fertile period. The woman was considered unclean after the menstrual period, so timing of intercourse was limited to the time of ovulation. This was certainly in accord with their injunction to be fertile and replenish the earth (Leviticus 15: 19–25).

STERILIZATION

As we have seen, some ancient societies practised ovariectomy on females and orchidectomy on males. In most cases such operations were done for contraceptive purposes, but sometimes religious and status motives were the reason. In ancient China, for instance, becoming a eunuch frequently led to power and influence at court.

At the present day as major contraceptive methods come under suspicion for one reason or another (the IUD, for example), more and more individuals are electing sterilization. The surgical techniques have become easier and less dangerous; for example, a tubal ligation or fulguration can be performed through a laparoscope with just a half inch sub-umbilical incision. A vasectomy is usually an office procedure. Morbidity is extremely low for both procedures and the convalescent time very short. One major disadvantage, however, is that for the usual case reversal is difficult or impossible. In cases of unrepairable tubes one can consider an *in vitro* fertilization as this procedure is becoming more accessible and easier to perform. The expense, which has been a major consideration in the past, although still high is becoming less important.

The acceptance of sterilization procedures has also changed. Hugo Hoogenboom of the Association for Voluntary Surgical Sterilization has said that in 1943 the availability of this method was practically non-existent. More and more women will now opt for sterilization rather than contend with the nuisance, side-effects and rare but potential dangers of oral and other traditional methods of contraception. As an illustration of the contemporary swing towards sterilization as a contraceptive method, the figures relating to the United States may be taken. The current incidence of surgical sterilization was given in an article in the US News and World Report (May 26, 1986). The 1986 figures indicate that 16.5 million Americans (58% female 42% male) have opted for surgery. This is up from 2.8 million in 1970. Two thirds of the vasectomies are done in the office and about 50% of tubal ligations take place on an out-patient basis. This increase is remarkable, but it must be remembered that the pill remains the first choice of women.

Previously most sterilizations were done on couples who had completed their families. Presently there is a disturbing new trend among younger women aged 20–24 which is up to 18% as compared to 13.4% 10 years ago. Dr Louise Tyrer of the Planned Parenthood Federation fears that many of the young women may have second thoughts. They opt for sterilization thinking that should they change their minds they could have a reversal procedure or *in vitro* fertilization. The former, however, is "chancy" and the latter time-consuming and expensive, despite the great strides in technique that have been made by specialists such as Patrick Steptoe, Alan Tronson and Georgiana and Howard Jones.

Attitudes towards these methods of birth control that we have reviewed have altered with the advent of the "Pill". An oral contraceptive that operates by regulating female hormone activity is a great advance, but it has been discovered that such intervention within the hormone area is not without risks; the gain in contraceptive efficacy has been huge, but short and long term hazards have had to be faced during the period of development of the "Pill". The next chapter considers this momentous scientific advance.

8

The Development of a
Contraceptive Pill

DISCOVERY OF THE HUMAN HORMONE SYSTEM

Germane to understanding the procreative function was the elucidation of the chemical communication system. William Harvey discovered the circulation of the blood in the early part of the 17th century. It took another 250 years before the chemical messenger system was discovered. The fact that the endocrine glands existed had been known much earlier from dissections but their function was not understood. As noted by Sir William Maddock Bayliss in 1924,

> "There are a large number of substances, acting powerfully in minute amounts, which are of great importance in physiologic processes. One class of these consists of the hormones, or chemical messengers, which are produced in a particular organ, pass into the blood current and produce effects in distant organs. They provide, therefore, for a chemical co-ordination of the activities of the organism, working side by side with that through the nervous system. The internal secretions, formed by ductless glands as well as by other tissues, belong to the class of hormones."

Professor Victor Medvei has pointed out that putting all of the pieces together was difficult because no single discipline was involved. Contributions were made in the fields of biochemistry, physiology, immunology, genetics, and molecular biology. It was only in the 1930s that the idea of an endocrine "orchestra" conducted by the pituitary gland came to fruition.

Many scientists contributed to the understanding of reproductive endocrinology. From early times it was recognized that castration had a marked effect on the body of man and animal alike. The bull was made tame, the swine fatter, etc. The term "sow gelder" was in common use by 1515.

Medvei points out that it is found in Burton's *The Anatomy of Melancholy*. One of the first observations on the effect of sow castration was reported by a French physician, Albert Puech. In an article in 1873, he reported uterine atrophy following early "spaying". Despite this, physicians were not intrigued enough to begin a study of ovarian endocrine function.

In 1889, Brown-Sequard began his attempts at rejuvenation by injecting testicular extracts. Villeneuve in Marseilles used the same method with ovarian extracts to control "hysteria" in women. Neither of these procedures was effective.

In the latter part of the 19th century, the histological anatomy of the various ovarian cells was studied. During the year 1897, R. H. J. Sobotta observed that the cells surrounding the ovum changed after ovulation. The preovulatory cells were termed granulosal and those after ovulation were called corpus luteum (yellow body), so-called because of the yellow appearance of the tissue. The endocrinological implications of his observations intrigued Auguste Pre'nant (1861–1927) and John Beard (1858–1924). They developed the Beard-Pre'nant hypothesis which was that the corpus luteum would suppress ovulation. These ideas were essential for the ultimate development of the pill.

Dr Ludwig Haberlandt (1885–1932) had the idea that successful birth control could be accomplished by hormonal manipulation. Ovarian transplant experiments had previously been done by Knauer in Vienna. Haberlandt's idea was that an animal could possibly be rendered infertile by transplanting the ovary of a pregnant animal into the body of a non-pregnant one. He was able to make five out of eight rabbits and three of eight guinea pigs infertile. The failures were due to tissue necrosis of the transplanted ovary. An even more farsighted idea was that oral ovarian extracts could possibly work. The initial experiments failed because the material supplied by the Merck Company came from non-pregnant ovaries.

At a meeting of the German Gynecological Society in Innsbruck in 1922 Haberlandt reported on his experiments. At the same meeting, Otfried Otto Fellner reported infertility following the injection of the lipid extract of corpus luteum. In the discussion, Fellner suggested that estrogen could possibly produce sterility. He was probably the first investigator to consider this use of estrogen. Following up on this idea, Fellner made up some estrogenic extract which he called "Feminin." When he used this material on 30 rabbits only three became pregnant and two developed pseudo-pregnancy. Haberlandt questioned the validity of Fellner's work, thus creating tension between the two scientists. Subsequently, Haberlandt admitted that estrogens might possibly be effective.

Progesterone had been isolated in 1905 by two students of Ludwig Fraenkel: Slotta, his son-in-law and Ruschig, another student. Scientists had at first no name for this hormone of the corpus luteum, some calling it "progestin", others suggesting "progesterone"; the latter designation was approved by most of the scientists at a meeting in London in 1935 and became the accepted name.

Unaware of the work of Haberlandt and Fellner, other investigators were experimenting with hormonal extracts. Makepeace, Weinstein and Friedman reported in 1937 that progesterone produced an anovulatory state in the rabbit. Gregory Pincus, also ignorant of the previous reports, was working with ovarian extracts.

DEVELOPMENT OF THE PILL

The first orally active progestational agent, 17α-ethyltestosterone, had been synthesized by a Schering scientist, Hans H. Inhoffen, just before the beginning of World War II. However, patient studies were apparently not done, and the preparation was not considered appropriate for clinical use. It was recognized that progesterone would inhibit ovulation, but extraction from animal sources was cumbersome, expensive and the yield poor. Large volumes of ovarian tissue were required to produce minute amounts of the extract. Thus, likely plant sources and the possibility of synthesization were investigated. The aim was to synthesize a chemical that would have the same biological effect as the naturally occurring female sex hormone (progesterone), and one, preferably, that could be administered orally. The original work was with steroid chemistry. Steroids are abundant in nature and are based on a chemical skeleton, a shorthand of which appears below:

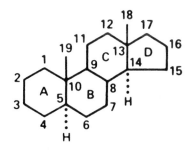

In the Australian sheep-rearing areas, it was noticed that when the animals were feeding in certain clover pastures the lamb production fell from as high as 80% to as low as 10%, but when the sheep were transferred to fresh fields reproduction rates returned to normal. Later, because of famine during the war, Dutch women ate tulip bulbs and became sterile. Russell Marker, an accomplished chemist and a far-sighted researcher had learned that in some plants a soap-like substance possessed the steroid (hormonal) nucleus. He had also noted that plants of the yam family, particularly the Mexican cabazadenegro, contained a high concentration of sapogenins (soap-forming elements).

Marker was an erratic genius, without whose discovery of plant steroids development of a contraceptive pill would not have occurred when it did.

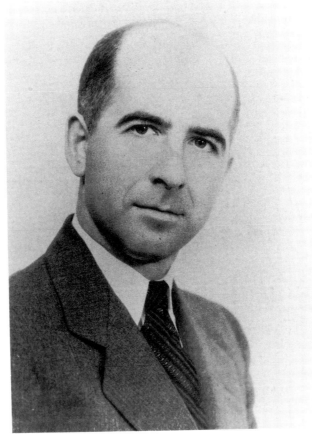

Russell Marker. (Photograph courtesy of Richard Edgren and Syntex Laboratory, Palo Alto, California)

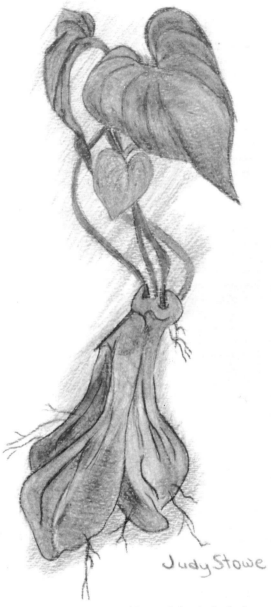

Mexican Yam. Cabazadenegro. (Courtesy of Syntex Laboratories Inc.)

Marker had attended the University of Maryland in the doctoral program in chemistry, but despite a brilliant thesis he did not receive the Ph.D degree because he refused to take a required course in physical chemistry which he considered boring and a waste of time. After leaving Maryland, he worked in industry for a short time and then spent six years at the Rockefeller Institute, from which he was offered an opportunity to do independent research at Pennsylvania State University for a very small stipend, augmented, apparently, by various grants. When the Parke-Davis Company, who had sponsored his earlier research, declined to fund further research, Marker left his position at Penn State in the middle of the school session and travelled to Mexico to begin research on the yam sapogenins. The yam nucleus is similar to that of cholesterol, but possesses a different side chain; it also resembles that of progesterone and Marker was able to degrade the E and F rings, thus producing progesterone.

Renting a crude laboratory, Marker manufactured 3000 grams of progesterone, having a value at the time of approximately $80.00 per gram. Marker then began to search for a chemical company with production capability. In the Mexico City phone book he found "Laboratories Hormona" listed and walked into their office with his sample of pure progesterone. It was not difficult to convince the two owners, Dr Emeric Somlo and Frederico Lehman, of the importance of his discovery. A new company was formed and named Syntex (Synthesis + Mexico). Marker obtained 40% of the shares. However, after only two years, following a dispute, Marker left and took with him his process. No patents had been taken out so within a short time the technique was widely copied. Marker's reaction was apparently to give up chemistry and research altogether. Dr Carl Djerassi, in his book *The Politics of Contraception*, comments that Marker should have been honored in many ways, but has been largely ignored. He did receive an award given in 1969 by the Mexican Chemical Society. When Dr Djerassi's book was published in 1979, Marker was 79 years of age and for the preceding 30 years he had devoted himself to commissioning Mexican-made silver artifacts. Gregory Pincus, in *The Control of Fertility* failed to mention Marker's contribution to the development of the pill. A similar lack of recognition was the inspiration for Major Sir Ronald Ross, a Nobel laureate for discovering the role of the mosquito in causing malaria, who wrote in 1917:

"Now twenty years ago
This day we found the thing;
With science and with skill
We found: then came the sting –

What we with endless labor won
The thick world scorned;
Not worth a word today —
Not worth remembering."

Meanwhile, back at Syntex, Somlo and Lehman had recruited Dr George Rosenkranz, a native of Switzerland. His training had been under Leonard Ruzicka, an early authority on steroid chemistry. The talented Rosenkranz had within two years learned the process of the manufacture of progesterone and in addition had been able to synthesize testosterone from the same Mexican yam.

In 1949, Dr Carl Djerassi was offered a position in research by Syntex. Working with Dr Rosenkranz, Dr Djerassi's forte was great knowledge of steroid chemistry. The manufacture of estrogen had been very difficult. The estrogen then in use was extracted from pregnant mares' urine. Using an aromatizing technique on the benzene ring, they were able to produce a synthetic hybrid which, it was hoped, would exhibit characteristics of both estrogen and progesterone. Their result proved to lack the expected qualities, but the technique became an essential chemical manipulation which would eventually lead to an orally active contraceptive pill.

Rosenkranz and Djerassi then were able to produce a crystalline 19 nor-progesterone by de-aromatization. Maximillian Ehrenstein in 1944 had transformed strophenthidin into 19-norprogesterone and this substance had proved by rabbit tests to have biological activity. The material was almost identical to natural progesterone except that a hydrogen atom rather than a methyl group was attached to the 10 position. The following diagrams illustrate the process:

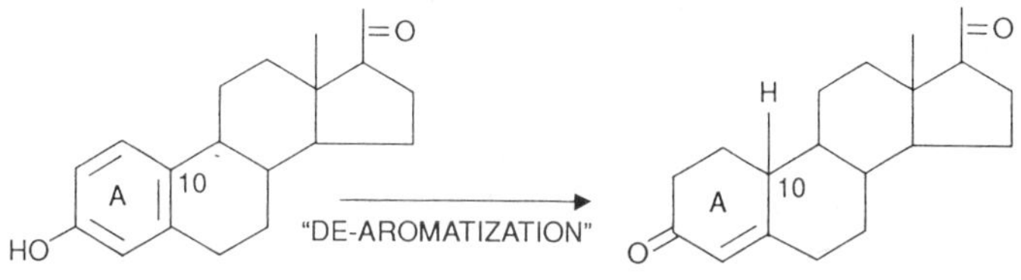

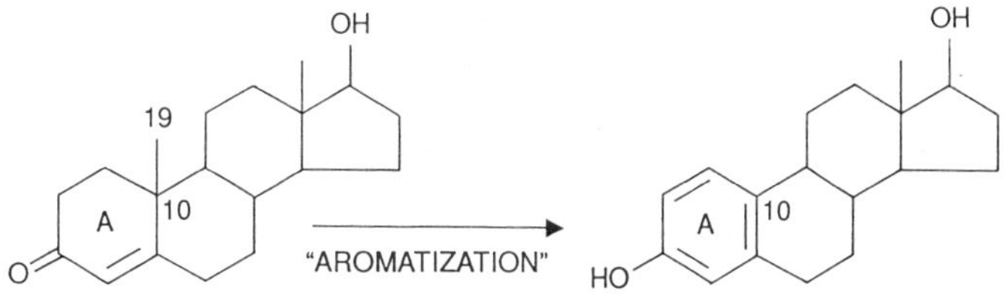

Although closely related, the sex steroids possess either female or male potential. The diagrams represented here are testosterone, the male sex hormone, and progesterone and estradiol, the two female hormones. The only difference between the male hormone testosterone and the female progesterone is the nature of the oxygen substituent at position 17. The only difference between the male hormone and the female estradiol is the benzene ring (A), an aromatic ring.

The Syntex team of Rosencranz, Djerassi and Miramontes removed the 19-methyl group, thus ending with ethisterone 19-norprogesterone. This material was sent to Roy Hertz at the National Cancer Institute, to Alexander

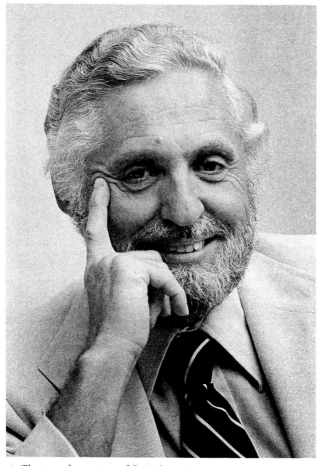

Carl Djerassi. (Photograph courtesy of R. A. Isaacs)

Lipschutz in Chile, to Gregory Pincus at the Worcester Foundation in Massachusetts, to Robert Greenblatt in Augusta, Georgia (a pioneer in steroid hormone therapy) and to Dr Edward Tyler in Los Angeles. Dr Tyler used this material in 1954 to treat menstrual and fertility problems.

Approximately a year later Frank Colton filed for a patent on the compound "norethynodrel", which was synthesized from unsaturated isomes of norethindrone and demonstrated similar clinical effects. Both norethindrone, a potent oral preparation synthesized by Djerassi, and norethynodrel were made commercially available in 1957.

REFLECTIONS ON THE DEVELOPMENT OF THE PILL

Much of the development of the pill was subject to the Baysean theorem, which was to revise probabilities when additional relevant information became available. There was certainly evidence of a unique particularity in the clinical behavior of steroids, and the development has the appearance of an evolutionary mosaic. Albert Schweitzer's ironic observation seems to apply in this case: "As we acquire more knowledge, things do not become more comprehensible but more mysterious".

This history of the development of the pill is incomplete for, as Professor Carl Djerassi points out in his book, some of the scientists have never told their story. Certain publications leave out vital information. As previously noted, Gregory Pincus in *The Control of Fertility*, failed to mention how the necessary steroid chemistry was discovered. The pharmacology of many, possibly most, valuable drugs has been elucidated by serendipity rather than predictability. An example is DDT, which was first synthesized for a purpose far removed from that of an insecticide. Since the time of Paul Ehrich (the father of chemotherapy), chemists have attempted to establish relationships between structure and biological activity.

In 1958, two years before the pill became a reality, Aldous Huxley wrote "Most of us chose birth control and immediately find ourselves confronted by a problem that is simultaneously a puzzle in physiology, pharmacology, sociology, psychology and even theology".

Biological truth is sometimes as hard to discover as it was for Menelaus when he tried to learn the truth from Proteus. Like the latter, science often confounds us by paradoxical behavior, but, as George Allen says, if we "allow it to run through its repertoire of possibilities, the truth will eventually emerge".

United States Patent Office

2,744,122
Patented May 1, 1956

1

2,744,122

Δ⁴-19-NOR-17α-ETHINYLANDROSTEN-17β-OL-3-ONE AND PROCESS

Carl Djerassi, Birmingham, Mich., and Luis Miramontes and George Rosenkranz, Mexico City, Mexico, assignors, by mesne assignments, to Syntex S. A., Mexico City, Mexico, a corporation of Mexico

No Drawing. Application November 12, 1952,
Serial No. 320,154

Claims priority, application Mexico November 22, 1951

4 Claims. (Cl. 260—397.4)

The present invention relates to cyclopentanophenanthrene derivatives and to a process for the preparation thereof.

More particularly the present invention relates to Δ⁴-19-nor-androsten-17β-ol-3-one compounds, having 17α-methyl or ethinyl substituents and to a process for producing these compounds.

In United States application of Djerassi, Rosenkranz and Miramontes, Serial Number 250,036, filed October 5, 1951, there is disclosed a novel process for the production of 19-norprogesterone. As set forth in this application, 19-norprogesterone has been found to be even stronger in its progestational effect than progesterone itself.

In accordance with the present invention, it has been found that the method described in detail in the aforementioned application may be applied to produce compounds of the androsten series, namely, Δ⁴-19-norandrosten-3,17-dione. By protecting the 3-keto group of this compound, as by the formation of a suitable enol ether as hereinafter set forth in detail and reacting the resultant 3 enol ether with suitable reagents, there may then be produced Δ⁴-19-nor-17α-methylandrosten-17β-ol-3-one or Δ⁴-19-nor-17α-ethinylandrosten-17β-ol-3-one. The first of these compounds exhibits more pronounced androgenic effects than its homologue methyltestosterone and the **second of these compounds exhibits more pronounced progestational effects than its homologue ethinyltestosterone.**

Certain of the novel compounds of the present invention may therefore be represented by the following structural formula:

In the above formula X is selected from the group consisting of C≡CH and CH₃.

Compounds as exemplified by the foregoing formula

2

may be produced in accordance with the process outlined by the following equation:

In the above equation R represents a lower alkyl radical, as for example methyl or ethyl, and R¹ represents a lower alkyl radical such as ethyl or methyl or a benzyl radical or any of the other groups which are customarily used as part of an enol ether customarily used for the protection of the 3-keto group of steroids. Thus, in the alternative rather than an alkyl or benzyl enol ether as shown benzyl thioenolethers may be utilized in the present reaction or other thioenolethers.

In practicing the process of the present invention, a suitable 3 lower alkyl ether as for example 3-methoxyestrone is dissolved in a suitable solvent such as anhydrous dioxane. Thereafter anhydrous liquid ammonia and an alkali metal, such as lithium or sodium metal, are added to the mechanically stirred solution. The stirring is continued for a short period, as for example one hour, and a quantity of ethanol is then added. When the reaction is complete and the blue color produced disappears, water is then added. The ammonia is then evaporated on a steam bath and the product collected with 2 L of water. Extraction with a suitable solvent, such as ether, and ethyl acetate followed by evaporation to dryness under vacuum, produced a yellow oil. The oil thus obtained was then dissolved in a suitable solvent, such as methanol, and refluxed with a mineral acid, such as hydrochloric acid, for approximately one hour. After purification, extraction and so forth, the product obtained was a yellow oil having an ultraviolet absorption maximum characteristic of a Δ⁴-3-ketone. The last-mentioned yellow oil was then oxidized as by adding chromic acid in acetic acid to a

Text for the copy of patent application for norethindrone by Carl Djerassi, November 22, 1951. It is interesting that contraception was not mentioned in the patent applications

Not only may science often appear paradoxical, scientists themselves occasionally play games. It is not often that a seriously written spoof appears in a first-class medical journal, but that is what occurred in 1965 in *The Canadian Medical Journal*. Dr Julius Greenstein's article entitled "Studies on a New, Peerless Contraceptive Agent: A Preliminary Final Report" described a new non-steroid drug called *armpitin*. The chemical structure was depicted as follows:

$$\langle\bigcirc\rangle \text{-NO-NO-NO-NO} \text{-----} \langle\bigcirc\rangle$$

The substance was to be applied to the axillary region as is done with deodorants. The effects described were that it increased the female libido and had a "tube-locking" effect on the male vas. The amazing thing is that serious scientists failed to recognize this tongue-in-cheek masterpiece for a spoof. Although an editorial in the same issue labelled the article for what it was, inquiries were still being received 14 years later. In answer to one letter, Dr Greenstein said that he was working on anti-armpitin nosedrops designed to protect the innocent exposed males.

The Sequential Pill

In 1961, Dr Robert Greenblatt came to the conclusion that hormonal replacement would be more physiological if estrogen was used in the first part of the cycle and progesterone in the latter part. The question was, "Would it work?" and the answer, "Yes". The sequential pill was subjected to the usual clinical trials and was approved by the Food and Drug Administration in 1965. Several years later, it was removed from the market because of a slightly higher failure rate and a slightly higher incidence of endometrial carcinoma.

Looking back, Dr Greenblatt felt that the estrogen dose should have been lower and the progestogen phase extended. He correctly pointed out that the sequential pill made more physiological sense than does the combination. The stoichiometric relationships are critical to the success and safety.

The Morning After Pill

In 1966, Morris and Van Wagener demonstrated that high doses of estrogen will prevent implantation of the fertilized egg. A survey of the literature revealed a pregnancy rate of 0.3% in 9,000 cases. Since then, the morning after pill has come to be used tens of thousands of times a year in countries such as Holland. Two tablets of a preparation such as Ovral twelve hours after unintended exposure to pregnancy is fully effective.

Long-acting Hormonal Contraceptives

A complete review of this subject is found in *Clinical Reproductive Endocrinology*, edited by Rodney P. Sherman, in Chapter 34, by Jan S. Fraser. Junkmann in 1953 discovered that the esterification of a progesterone alcohol resulted in a preparation that had long-lasting effect when injected. Shortly thereafter, in 1958, other long-acting progestogens were discovered, i.e., norethisterone oethanate by Junkmann and Welzel and depomedroxyprogesterone acetate by Babcock *et al.* In 1967 the Upjohn Company applied for approval from the Food and Drug Administration to market the latter drug under the name of Depo Provera. A history of this as it concerns contraception is detailed elsewhere.

Long-acting hormones have been used to control animal populations, which may increase to the point that the ecological balance is disturbed. In the Etosha National Park in Namibia in Africa, when the numbers of lions exceeded the ideal level, drastic measures were needed and Dr Hu Berry and Dr Jock Orford implanted time-release capsules containing the hormones in anesthesized females.

The Safety of the Pill

There is a natural reluctance inherent in the thinking of men and women which causes them to fear any tampering with natural body functions, or, for that matter, with abnormal functions. Many initially rejected the use of insulin in the treatment of diabetes even after Banting and Best had demonstrated its safety and life-saving properties. It is even easier to understand reluctance to change other normal endocrine functions.

When the first reports of possible cardiovascular complications associated with the pill were publicized, there was a "stampeding effect" on the part of patient and physician alike. Reluctance to accept the new has been a common trait of physicians even to modern times. Many have, perhaps wisely, followed the dictum of Alexander Pope, whose caution was "Be not the first to lay the old aside. Nor the last by whom the new is tried". It is, and has always been, in the patient's best interest to weigh benefit and safety on the one hand and danger on the other. Kenneth Ryan once said that there are no risk-free options in life. One would add, however, that excessive caution can be dangerous also. Perhaps Reah Tannahill's conclusion was correct when she said that the medical profession was as conservative as the women who depended upon them.

It is not the purpose of this writer to discuss the reported dangers of the pill, except to offer the following: (1) the currently used low-dose combination pill is considerably safer than the original higher-dose one, and (2) one must balance the risk of pregnancy with those of any preventive measure.

Dr Daniel Mishell states that a review of the literature shows that in the 22 years since the availability of oral contraceptives there has been no increase in the incidence of cancer of the breast, uterine body or cervix. If one discontinues the pill and becomes pregnant immediately, the incidence of spontaneous abortion is not increased, contrary to the belief of some.

There does appear to be a slightly increased risk of myocardial infarction, although the absolute risk is very low. In fact, the overall rate of death from heart attacks in the 20–45 age group has decreased in the past 15 years for both men and women. Another fact involved in epidemiological evaluations is whether or not existing risk factors are present, i.e. hypertension, vascular problems and smoking.

The length of time the pill is used has been a concern. Initially, it was felt that the pill user should get off the medication after three to five years. Recent data indicate that this is not necessary.

Another fear has been that if young girls were started on the pill the estrogen component would hasten closure of the epiphysis, thus resulting in reduced height or permanent changes in the hypothalamic pituitary-ovarian axis. Neither of these concerns has proved to be true. As with all drugs, some side-effects are experienced but a discussion of these is not deemed germane.

An evaluation of the debate was eloquently discussed by Richard Edgren, a pioneer in the development of oral contraception. In an article, "Erewhon: The Destination of Retrospection", Dr Edgren calls attention to retrospective evaluation. He begins by quoting Yale statistician Alvar Feinstein who labelled this type of analysis "Cohot Trohoc."

> "Since millions of women are employing oral contraceptives now and have used them in the past, oral contraceptive patients will suffer from virtually all known diseases and will die from all possible causes, from accidents to zoonoses. Improper causal relations will be assigned, and we will be unable to give direct, simple answers to demands like, 'Prove the oral contraceptives don't cause prostatic cancer, or an increase in snake bite.' If the past is an augury of the future, many Trohocians will have no qualms about damning drugs for the flimsiest of reasons."

Mark Twain said that fluid prejudice is the ink with which all history is written.

According to Jan S. Fraser, the public, the politicians and the consumer groups expect and demand that a drug be 100% safe and 100% effective as well. There is nothing in the world pharmacopeia that even approximates this Utopian ideal. Dr Fraser cites an article in the *Lancet* which concludes with these words by Sir Douglas Black: "certainly not absolutely safe, which would imply that it was totally ineffective, but as safe as reasonable precautions by all concerned can make it, consistent with appropriate therapeutic benefit". It has been pointed out by many authors that currently available methods of birth control, i.e., the pill, IUD, condom, diaphragm and even abortion constitute less of a threat to life than pregnancy and childbirth.

The pill is extremely effective and actually very safe, particularly when the new low-dose regimens are used. To compare the noxious, dangerous and ineffective nostrums used in the past with the pill is like comparing a plow horse to Pegasus.

Needless to say, there was much lay interest in the development of the pill and, as Lester King has pointed out, lay interest can distort our perspective. In this endeavor there was the ego of the scientist, the economic risk for the pharmaceutical industry, the moral position of the church and the hopes and fears of the prospective patient.

Innovation seems to be more difficult the more one is trained in the traditional. In the development of the pill, many scientists had to unlearn and relearn; as Shakespeare said in *As You Like It*, each one had to "unmuzzle your (his) wisdom".

According to the American College of Obstetrics and Gynecology Newsletter of January, 1987, Dr Christopher Tietze was recognized for revolutionizing physician views concerning the safety and efficiency of available contraceptive methods. Dr Tietze died in 1984 at age 75. His papers are being edited by his widow and will be published by Springer-Verlag, New York.

IMPORTANT FIGURES IN THE DEVELOPMENT OF THE PILL

The persons most responsible for the development, clinical testing and marketing of the first oral contraceptive were Gregory Pincus, Min Cheuh Chang, John Rock and Celso Garcia. Drs Pincus and Chang were research scientists and Drs Rock and Garcia were clinicians. The association of these men was to prove a very productive one.

Dr Gregory Pincus is known as the "father of the pill". While he deserves much credit, the accolade could go to others, for example Makepeace, who reported in 1937 that progesterone could prevent ovulation in the rabbit, or further back, Haberlandt and Fellner, both of whom observed that both estrogen and progesterone could have that effect. The author's nominee would be Dr Russell Marker, who extracted a potent, orally active progesterone from the Mexican yam. One should also mention Dr Carl Djerassi and the Syntex chemists. Nevertheless, the Pincus name is synonymous with the pill.

Professor Pincus was a biologist at the Worcester Foundation in Shrewsbury, Massachusetts. Chance provided him with an introduction to Margaret Sanger at a dinner party. Mrs Sanger expressed the hope that an effective oral preparation could be found. Dr Pincus promised that he would "look into it".

After receiving a grant from the Planned Parenthood Federation of America, he was able to obtain some progesterone, thanks to Dr Marker's work. Dr John Rock had previously used small doses of injectable progesterone to treat infertility patients. His theory was that if ovarian function could be temporarily put at rest, cessation of treatment could result in a rebound of ovarian function and an increased chance for pregnancy.

In order to further assess the effect of progestagens on ovulation, Dr Pincus recruited Dr Celso Ramon Garcia in the United States and Edris Rice Wray and Manuel Paniagua of Puerto Rico. Clinical trials indicated that 20 days of hormone treatment would prevent ovulation and that this was apparently harmless to other organ systems. The studies began in 1956. By 1960 the Food and Drug Administration approved the marketing of Enovid by G. D. Searle Company and Ortho Novum by Ortho Pharmaceuticals in 1962.

The incidence of side-effects and serious complications was very low. It was soon learned that ovulation could be prevented by much lower doses than that in the original pill, so that the current preparations are as effective and are much safer.

Dr Rock became convinced that the hormonal suppression of ovulation was vastly different in a moral sense from the use of barrier or spermicidal methods. He felt that the Roman Catholic church should allow use of this method. His story and case is eloquently told in his book, *The Time Has Come*.

Von Baeyer, in his book, *Rainbows, Snowflakes, and Quarks*, uses the word *themata* to describe the way of thinking in physics: "Themata are unspoken premises, prejudices, assumptions based in intuition. They are persistent motifs or subconscious biases that guide the thinking of even the most theoretical scientist". The term seems a good one to characterize those "greats" who elucidated the mysteries of steroid chemistry.

Gregory Pincus

Gregory ("Goodie") Pincus was born in Woodbine, New Jersey, in 1903. Both his maternal and paternal forebears were Russian Jews. Farming was the family occupation. Gregory's father was a teacher and editor of a farm journal. One uncle was Dean of the agriculture school at Rutgers University. "Goodie" wanted to be a farmer but his father discouraged him because of the economic hardships suffered by many in agriculture. Gregory graduated from Cornell in 1924 with a B.S. degree in biology. He was much interested in genetics because of his own inherited color blindness.

One of the country's leading geneticists was Dr William Castle at Harvard. Pincus found the academic atmosphere at Harvard to be very congenial. He earned his M.S. and Sc.D. degrees in 1927. He then left for Europe in order to study at Cambridge University and at the Kaiser Wilhelm Institute. By

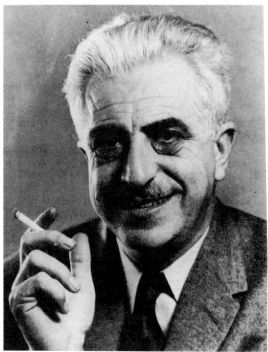

Dr Gregory Pincus

this time, he was firmly committed to reproductive physiology. He returned to Havard to work under William Crozier. His associate and collaborator was Hudson Hoagland. In 1938 he was given a year's leave of absence and prior to his departure he was told that his appointment at Harvard would not be renewed. Pincus felt that the current anti-Semitism was the reason. He moved his family to Cambridge, England, but it was soon apparent that the holocaust was on the way, and he became anxious to return to the United States. His friend, Hudson Hoagland, then at Clark University, was able to secure for him a non-paying appointment as visiting professor of zoology. His Cambridge friend, Baron Rothschild, provided a stipend. Later, Hoagland and a New York businessman, Henry Illeson, raised funds for him to be an independent researcher in Worcester, Massachusetts. Subsequently, through funding by grants from the Rockefeller and Macy Foundations, he was able to establish the Worcester Foundation. It was during his directorship that Margaret Sanger encouraged him to work on birth control.

Min Cheuh Chang

Min Cheuh Chang was recruited to work at the Worcester facility. He was a brilliant investigator but his lack of fluency in English was a handicap. Chang began his work on progesterone in 1951. His careful experiments and impeccable data did much to further development of hormonal contraception. Much honor is due him.

John Rock

As a Harvard professor and as an authority on infertility, Dr John Rock had used progesterone to suppress ovarian function. He had found that when ovarian function was suppressed for a time and then suppression ended, a rebound resulted in ovulation. When Pincus sought to recruit John Rock, who was a Roman Catholic, Margaret Sanger felt that he had made a poor choice. She later came to recognize that Dr Rock was his own man. There are moments and early experiences that have a profound effect in later life. One such experience was related by Dr Rock. A curate of his parish church asked the boy, John, to accompany him on a visit to a "poor farm". While driving there, Father Finnick suddenly said, "John, always stick to your conscience; never let anyone else keep it for you". He let that remark soak in, then added, "And I mean *anyone* else". Perhaps Father Finnick recognized something unusual about John Rock: that he would be a man of conviction, tempered by a concern for his fellow man and the moral code of the

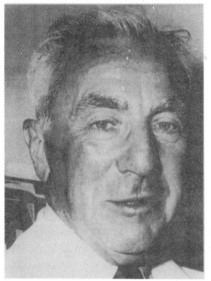
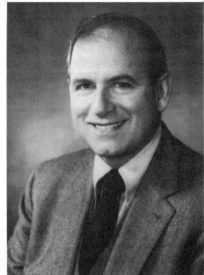

John Rock (Courtesy of Dr C.R. Garcia)   Celso Garcia

Christian faith.

His work on the hormonal suppression of ovulation persuaded Dr Rock that this was a method of birth control that could be acceptable to the Roman Catholic church. There was no suspicion that it might cause abortion. His book, *The Time has Come*, presented his arguments to those of his faith.

Celso Ramon Garcia

Dr Garcia was born in New York City in 1921. He received his M.D. degree at the New York State University of Medicine at Brooklyn. His internship was served at the Norwegian Lutheran Hospital in Brooklyn. Following a residency in pathology, he became a research fellow in obstetrics and gynecology at Cumberland Hospital. He was next assigned Assistant Professor at San Juan City Hospital where he conducted clinical trials with the new oral contraceptive. Following this, he was made Director of the training programme at the Worchester Foundation. From 1965 to the present he has been Professor of obstetrics and gynecology at the University of Pennsylvania Hospital in Philadelphia.

Dr Garcia is highly intelligent, an excellent researcher and teacher, a prolific writer and a very nice and warm person.

Conclusion: Population Control and the Future

In his *Reconsiderations*, Professor Toynbee summarizes the course of civilizations. Citing J. A. Mason's *Courses in the Age of Civilizations*, he notes that all civilizations have developed along more or less identical lines. He describes this process as similar to a tragic drama in three acts. The first is described as the golden age, characterized by the development of agriculture. The second act is characterized by pressures caused by increasing population, and the third by contending states resorting to military conflicts. Toynbee asks whether we can liberate ourselves from this grim scenario. Pessimistically he predicts that man is not likely to use advanced technology wisely, and he sees as the only hope the influence of spiritual virtues of imagination, wisdom, self-control and, above all, good intent. "These are the keys to man's destiny." The challenge of over-population, characteristic of Act II, is very much with us now. How effective will our response be?

The severity of the problem faced by the modern world is difficult to grasp and difficult to exaggerate. For a number of reasons associated with its success, the human race seems progressively to have learned to escape from the natural controls over population which regulate other forms of life, and we now appear to be on a mad and threatening career of multiplication. Developing control over the environment and attention to individual welfare have, broadly speaking, made the average human life viable for more years, but conditioning, based on earlier race experience presumably, continues to prompt a fertility that once offered security but now threatens disaster. Konrad Lorenz in his *Civilized Man's Eight Deadly Sins* expressed the predicament very well. "All those gifts that have sprung from man's deep insight into the nature of his surroundings — the progress of his technology, his chemical and medical sciences, everything that seems most likely to relieve human suffering — works in a horrible and paradoxical way toward the destruction of mankind, and humanity threatens to do what living systems almost never do, namely to suffocate in itself".

139

The question now is whether the human race is capable of sufficient collective consciousness and will to act to control population and permit the benefits flowing from the ascent of man to be enjoyed by the race as a whole. Will we be able to achieve sufficient unity of awareness so that a population disaster is turned away? Many express their doubts; Professor H. Brown of California Institute of Technology in 1969 excellently described the crossroads predicament. Population increase, he believes, underlies an instability which take all forms.

> "It might well turn out that humanity will not be able to extricate itself from its present precarious situation. Increasing population pressures, rising rates of population growth and decreasing per capita availability of food in the poorer regions of the world, a widening gap between the rich countries and the poor, a restlessness in the poorer countries stimulated in part by the spreading realization that from a technological point of view they too could lead lives free of deprivation — all these factors breed political chaos, violence, and unreasoning actions which threaten nations and people. Even a casual survey of current trends indicates that people in the poorer countries will probably be even hungrier a decade from now than they are today; that improvement in economic conditions will take place so slowly that the average individual will not notice much change for the better during his lifetime, that internal political chaos in these areas will increase rapidly; that political differences among richer nations, when coupled with the tribulations of the poorer ones, can lead to major wars and eventually to the downfall in industrial civilization.
>
> At the same time it is becoming increasingly evident that modern science and technology have given man unprecedented power. We are clearly able from a technological point of view to feed adequately a population considerably larger than that of today, to control its growth, to educate, clothe, and house it. Indeed, we can create a world in which all people, if they wish, can lead free and abundant lives"*.

There seems no doubt that population control is perhaps the major challenge to human destiny in the next one or two hundred years. What must be done?

Political circumstances suggest that an unacceptable population control mechanism, a terrible brother to traditional natural disasters such as famine, earthquake, volcano and epidemic, could be at hand to cull the species — or, at worst, eliminate it. Nuclear war, following which only "fit" species such as the cockroach and other insects might survive, is a possible population control device that should, in its horror, enforce purposeful thinking and action along other lines. Laboriously engineered international

From "Food and the Energy Transition" by H. Brown. In *Fertility and Family Planning: A World View* (1969). S.J. Behrman, L. Corsa Jr. and R. Freeman. (Ann Arbor: U. of Michigan Press)

good faith must restrain the potential for nuclear war and, similarly, international good will and the flow of information are prerequisites for the acceptance of ambitious population control strategies. Changes in awareness must take place both in the Third World where the birthrate among the deprived is so high, and in the developed countries, even though population growth there is not an immediate problem.

Governments and peoples of the Third World need to be brought to believe that population control is not a device on the part of developed nations whereby existing privilege is perenniated. Many suspicions continue concerning the motives of developed nations in pressing population control on ironically termed "developing" nations. Might not, for instance, population control be favored because it will effectively hold back a wave of racially inferior human beings? Perhaps population control is a means of controlling and inhibiting economic growth, and with it political power and independence? These considerations of international relations are, of course, over and above any religious or cultural imperatives that bear upon the topic.

We can be sure that Third World countries will not be persuaded by words alone. Affluent and stable countries will be required to *do* things, not just prescribe. Aid, for instance, must be targeted to benefit countries as a whole, not just client élites. Multinational companies must submit to some regimen that prevents them from negotiating (through strength)

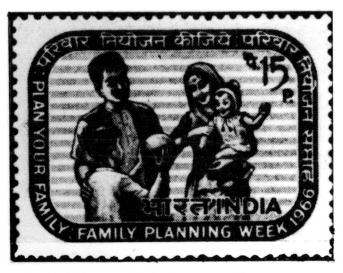

Indian stamp issued in furtherance of Family Planning promotion "agreements" that have a distorting and damaging effect on struggling host countries. Pharmaceutical companies, for instance, must not be found supplying new, complex and inappropriate drugs to medical services that are short of aspirin and swabs. A responsible attitude toward the use of the unreplenishable resources of the planet needs to be developed and publicized and, in conjunction with this, advanced societies are more likely to be persuasive over population control matters if they can show that the concept of "enough" can have some meaning within affluent circumstances. In such ways are economic, political and social factors associated with the task of leading the peoples of the Third World to see the advantage of and accept population control.

International understanding and action are required to further the cause but, equally, the influence of domestic cultural and religious outlooks need to be taken into account. Such policy is not invariably in force at present. Whether the People's Republic of China will succeed in its attempt to cut the Gordian knot by forbidding couples to have more than a single child is yet to be seen. This radical policy, which seems wholly to ignore traditional attitudes, is not, however, so authoritarian and inflexible as it might appear. The local community (or commune) provides supportive counselling and, where necessary, it also provides sanctions such as the withdrawal of housing privileges. Deep beliefs in the Third World about gender roles, the meaning and mechanics of the sex act, the significance of children, the role of the extended family are sometimes barely within reach of rational, scientific challenge, and policy encouraging birth control must negotiate sensitively and patiently with these forces. Neither the blatant one-off bribe of a transistor radio nor intent technical explanation can be expected effectively to override deep traditional convictions. Perhaps the way to success in this area lies with the role played by the educated, mediating class in Third World societies — people who have assimilated a wide perspective and yet can negotiate in an understanding way with fellow citizens who are unquestioningly under the influence of traditional values. Such "enlightened" people face huge tasks of many sorts, and they undergo abnormal stress on account of the range of values they have to try to integrate so as to retain personal stability and effectiveness.

The future, we must hope, will show movement towards safer, more effective and more easily administered birth control methods. To achieve this, science will need to move forward with as little encumbrance as possible. Funding needs to be adequate, both from government and private sources. The role of the pharmaceutical companies is a crucial but difficult one. Profits have to be appropriately allocated as between the investing citizen and future research, and unlike some other corporate businesses, pharmaceutical companies accept a notable burden of responsibility to the community. Self-regulation and market forces provide some guidelines, but government agencies, especially as regards the international and Third World context, need to contribute assistance and perspective. Pharmaceutical companies must continue to try to show care and concern, and the complex relation between companies, drug administration agencies, consumer groups and animal rights organisations must be watched and adjusted by reasoned discourse.

Scientific research, in birth control as in other fields, has increasingly to justify itself to a far from quiescent public. While scientific manipulation of man and his environment can be shown, in some cases, to have been damaging, the need for continuing innovation is generally undisputed. In the field of contraception scientists must attend to public opinion so that a reasonable level of risk in connection with innovation is rationally tolerated. All currently known contraceptive measures have their dangers and failures, and further development cannot be exempt from such. After all, pregnancy and childbirth offer significant risk, as does the use of automobiles...

It is now being realized how early research into hormone contraceptives was limited by dependence on animal models. As Professor Djerassi and others have pointed out, the commonly used beagle bitch has lead to some misleading conclusions especially in connection with safety factors. Canine reproductive cycles are vastly different from that of the human. In spite of all past problems, we may reasonably expect continuing advances, perhaps especially in relation to contraception for the male.

This book comes to a conclusion by considering contraception within the modern world context, and the problem of over population certainly compels attention. But we should not willingly lose sight of the individual experience in relation to contraception. So much to do with the quality of individual lives, their happiness or misery, debility or well-being, fulfilment or entrapment depends, world-wide, on the availability or otherwise of contraception.

Select Reading List

1. Allen, G. (1980). *The Importance of Past Meditations on the Authority of Tradition*. (New York: State University of New York Press)

2. Aquinas, St. Thomas. *Summa Theologica*, translated by Dominican fathers. In: *Great Books of the Western World*. (Chicago: University of Chicago press, 1952)

3. Ardrey, R. (1970). *The Social Contract*. (New York: Atheneum Press)

4. Ardrey, R. (1966). *The Territorial Imperative*. (New York: Atheneum Press)

5. Barker, G.H. (1981). *Your Search for Fertility*. (New York: William Morrow)

6. Behrman, S.J., Corsa, L. and Friedman, R. (eds.) (1969). *Fertility and Family Planning*. (Ann Arbor: University of Michigan Press)

7. Benet, W.R. (ed.) (1948). *The Readers Encyclopedia of World Literature*. (New York: Thomas Y. Crowell Company)

8. Biedermann, H. *Medicena Magica*, In: *The Classics of Medicine*. (1986). (Birmingham, Alabama: Gryphon, Inc.)

9. Bonar, J. (1966). *Malthus and his Work: Reprints of Economic Classics*. (New York: Augustus M. Kelley) (First edition: Frank Cass & Co., London, 1885)

10. Bowen, C.D. (1963). *Francis Bacon: the Temper of a Man*. (Boston: Little Brown & Co.)

11. Briffault, R. (1927). *The Mothers: a Study of Sentiments and Institutions*. (New York: Macmillan & Company)

12. Brown, H. and Leech, M. (1927). *Roundsman of the Lord*. (New York: A & C Boni Publishers)

13. Bullock, A. and Stallybrass, O. (eds.) (1977). *The Harper Dictionary of Modern Thought*. (New York: Harper & Row)

14. Burton, R. (1621). *The Anatomy of Melancholy* (Ann Arbor: Michigan State University Press, L. Babb, ed., 1963)

15. Castiglioni, A. *A History of Medicine*, trans. E.B. Krumbhoar. (New York: Alfred A. Knopf, 1941)

16. Cavendish, R. (ed.) (1980). *Mythology: an Illustrated Encyclopedia*. (New York: Rizzoli)

17. Cook, R.C. (1971). *Human Fertility: the Modern Dilemma*. (Westport, Connecticut: Greenwood Publishing)

18. Cousins, N. (1983). *The Healing Heart*. (New York: W. W. Norton)

19. DeKruif, P. (1930). *Microbe Hunters*. (New York: Blue Ribbon Books)

20. *Dictionary of Scientific Biography*, Vol. 9. (1980). (New York: Charles Scribner's Sons)

21. Djerassi, C. (1981). *The Politics of Contraception*. (San Francisco: W.H. Freeman)

22. Durant, W. and Durant, A. (1967). *Rousseau and Revolution*. (New York: Simon & Schuster)

23. Durant, W. (1953). *The Story of Civilization, Vol. V, The Renaissance.* (New York: Simon & Schuster)
24. Durant, W. and Durant, A. (1945). *Rousseau and Revolution*, Vol. XI (New York: Simon & Schuster)
25. Durant, W. (1945). *The Story of Philosophy.* (New York: Simon & Schuster)
26. Eliot, C. (ed.) (1980). *The Harvard Classics, Vol. I: Sacred Writings.* (Danbury, Connecticut: Gryphon Enterprises)
27. *Encyclopaedia Britannica, Vol. II.* (1973). (Chicago: William Benton Publisher)
28. *Encyclopaedia Britannica, Vol. XI.* (1979). (Chicago: William Benton Publisher)
29. Finch, B.E. and Green, H. (1963). *Contraception through the Ages.* (London: Owen Publishing Company)
30. Frazer, J.A. (1911). *The Golden Bough: a Study in Magic and Religion.* (London: Macmillan)
31. Friedan, B. (1963). *The Female Mystique.* (New York: Dell Publishing)
32. Gardner, J. (1978). *The Life and Times of Chaucer.* (New York: Vintage Books Division of Random House)
33. Garrison, F.H. (1960). *An Introduction to the History of Medicine.* (Philadelphia: W.B Saunders Company)
34. Gay, P. (1966). *Great Ages of Man: Age of Enlightenment.* (New York: Time Life Books)
35. Gillespie, C.D. (ed.) (1980). *Dictionary of Scientific Biography.* (New York: Charles Scribner's Sons)
36. Graham, H. (1951). *Eternal Eve: The History of Gynecology and Obstetrics.* (New York: Doubleday & Company)
37. Green, S. (1971). *The Curious History of Contraception.* (New York: St Martin's Press)
38. Greenblatt, R.B. (1985). *Search the Scriptures: Modern Medicine and Biblical Personages.* (Carnforth, Lancs., U.K.: Parthenon Publishing)
39. Gupte, P. (1984). *The Crowded Earth: People and the Politics of Population.* (New York: W.W. Norton Company)
40. Hajnal, J. European marriage patterns in perspective. In: Glass, D.V. and Eversley, D.E.C., (eds.) (1964). *Population in History.* (London: Arnold Press)
41. Handler, P. (ed.) (1970). *Biology and the Future of Man.* (London: Oxford University Press)
42. Hardin, G. (ed.) (1969). *Population Evolution and Birth Control,* 2nd ed. (San Francisco: W. H. Freeman & Co.)
43. Himes, N.E. (1963). *Medical History of Contraception.* (New York: Gamut Press, Inc.)
44. Hixson, J. (1976). *The Patchwork Mouse.* (New York: Anchor Press)
45. Hugo, V. *Les Misérables.* (New York: Fawcett Publishing, 1979)
46. Hutchins, R.M. and Adler, M.J. (eds.) (1963). Gateway to the great books. In: *Encyclopaedia Britannica.* (Chicago: William Benton Publisher)
47. Huxley, A. (1965). *Brave New World Revisited.* (New York: Harper & Row)
48. Jordan, L. (ed.) (1979). *The New York Manual of Style and Usages.* (New York: Times Books)
49. Karlen, A. (1984). *Napoleon's Glands and other Ventures in Biohistory.* (Boston: Little, Brown & Company)
50. Khayyam, O. *Rubaiyat.* (New York: Grosset & Dunlap, Galahad Books)
51. Kistner, R.W. (1968). *The Pill: Facts and Fallacies about Today's Oral Contraceptives.* (New York: Delacort Press)

52. Leach, G. (1970). *The Biocrats.* (New York: McGraw-Hill)

53. Lewin, R. (1987). *Bones of Contention.* (New York: Simon & Schuster)

54. Lissner, J. (1962). *The Silent Past,* trans. J. Maxwell Brownjohn. (New York: G.P. Putmans Sons)

55. Lorenz, K. (1974). *Civilized Man's Eight Deadly Sins.* (New York: Harcourt Brace Jovanovich

56. Lorenz, K (1973) *Behind the Mirror: a Search for a Natural History of Human Knowledge.* (New York: Harcourt Brace Jovanovich)

57. Lorenz, K. (1966). *On Aggression.* (New York: Harcourt Brace Jovanovich)

58. Lyons, A.S. and Petrucelli, R.J. (1978). *Medicine, an Illustrated History.* (New York: Henry N. Abrams)

59. Maisel, A.Q. (1965). *The Hormone Quest.* (New York: Random House)

60. Masters, J. (1969). *Casanova.* (New York: Bernard Geis Associates)

61. Medawar, P.B. and Medawar, J.S. (1977). *The Life Science: Current Ideas of Biology.* (New York: Harper & Row)

62. Medvei, V.C. (1984). *A History of Endocrinology.* (Lancaster: MTP Press)

63. Mendelson, E., Swazey, J.P. and Taviss, J. (1971). *Human Aspects of Biomedical Innovation.* (Cambridge, Massachusetts: Harvard University Press)

64. Milton, J. (1667). *Paradise Lost.* In: *The Complete Poems of Milton.* (1980). Eliot, C.W. (ed.) (Danbury, Connecticut: Grolier Enterprises Corp.)

65. Milton J. Introduction to "Samson Agonistes". In: *The Complete Poems of Milton.* (1980). Eliot, C.W. (ed.) (Danbury, Connecticut: Grolier Enterprises Corp.)

66. Moyer, D.L, (ed.) (1968). *Progress in Conception Control.* (Philadelphia: J. B. Lippincott)

67. Noonan, J.T. (1966). *Contraception: a History of its Treatment by the Catholic Theologians and Canonists.* (Cambridge, Massachusetts: The Belknap Press of Harvard University Press)

68. Packard, V. (1968). *The Sexual Wilderness.* (New York: David McKay)

69. Panati, C. (1987). *Extraordinary Origins of Everyday Things.* (New York: Harper & Row)

70. Pincus, G. (1965). *The Control of Fertility.* (New York: Academic Press)

71. Raffel, B. (1978). (trans.) *Beowulf.* (New York: New American Library)

72. Reed, J. (1978). *The Birth Control Movement and American Society: from Private Vice to Public Virtue.* (Princeton, New Jersey: Princeton University Press)

73. Richie, P. (1978). *Daily Life in the World of Charlemagne.* Trans. J.A. McNamara. (Pittsburg: University of Pennsylvania Press)

74. Robertson, P. (1982). *The Book of Firsts.* (New York: Bramhall House Division of Clarkson N. Potter, Inc.)

75. Rock, J. (1963). *The Time Has Come.* (New York: Alfred A. Knopf)

76. Rosebery, T. (1971). *Microbes and Morals.* (New York: The Viking Press)

77. Rouse, A.L. (1974). *Sex and Society in Shakespeare's Age.* (New York: Charles Scribner's Sons)

78. Russell, B. (1945). *A History of Western Philosophy.* (New York: Simon & Schuster)

79. Shaw, H. (1987). *Dictionary of Problem Words and Expressions.* (New York: McGraw Hill)

80. Shearman, R.P. (ed.) (1985). *Clinical Reproductive Endocrinology.* (London: Churchill Livingstone)

81. Sigerist, H.E. (1960). *On the Sociology of Medicine.* (New York: M. D. Publications)

82. Sindermann, C.J. (1984). *Winning the Games Scientists Play.* (New York: Plenum Press)

83. Smith, A. (1975). *The Human Pedigree.* (Philadelphia: J. B. Lippincott Co.)
84. Taylor, G.R. (1968). *The Biological Time Bomb.* (Cleveland, Ohio: New American Library)
85. Thomas, L. (1974). *The Lives of a Cell.* (New York: Viking Press)
86. Tolbot, C.H. (1967). *Medicine in Medieval England.* (New York: American Elsevier Publishing Co.)
87. Toynbee, A.J. (1986). *An Historian's Approach to Religion.* (New York: Oxford University Press)
88. Toynbee, A.J. (1961). *A Study of History: Vol.XII: Reconsideration.* (New York: Oxford University Press)
89. Toynbee, A.J. (1954). *A Study of History, Vols. I-VIII.* (New York: Oxford University Press)
90. Vogt, W. (1948). *The Road to Survival.* (New York: W. Sloane Associates)
91. Von Baeyer, H.C. (1987). *Snowflakes, Rainbows and Quarks.* (New York: McGraw Hill)
92. Weisman, G. (1987). *They All Laughed at Christopher Columbus: Tales of Medicine and the Art of Discovery.* (New York: Time-Life Books Division of Random House)
93. Williams, K. (1958). *Jonathan Swift and the Age of Compromise.* (University of Kansas Press)
94. Wood, C. and Suitters, B. (1970). *A Fight for Acceptance. A History of Contraception.* (Aylesbury, Bucks, U.K.: MTP Press)

Index

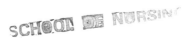